From There To Here

From There To Here

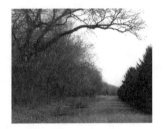

a breast cancer journey

by Diane Davies

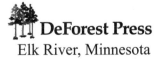
DeForest Press
Elk River, Minnesota

Permission gratefully acknowledge for the following:
Reprinted poems from the books *Hurdles Are For Jumping* and *Once Upon A Shooting Star*, as well as original poems, all written by Carolyn Salter.
Quote on page 39 from *Ask the Doctor: Breast Cancer*, copyright © 1997 by Vince Friedewald, M.D. Used by permission of Andrews and McMeel. All rights reserved.

Scripture quotations are taken from the *Holy Bible*, New Living Translation, copyright © 1996. Used by permission of Tyndale House Publishers, Inc., Wheaton, Illinois 60189. All rights reserved.

Published by:
DeForest Press
P.O. Box 154
Elk River, MN 55330 USA
www.DeForestPress.com
Toll-free: 877-441-9733
Richard DeForest Erickson, Publisher
Shane Groth, President

Cover design by Linda Walters, Optima Graphics, Appleton, WI

ISBN 1-930374-18-6

Printed in the United States of America
09 08 07 06 05   5 4 3 2 1

Library of Congress Cataloging-in-Publication Data

Davies, Diane, 1948-
  From there to here : a breast cancer journey / by Diane Davies.
    p. cm.
  ISBN 1-930374-18-6
  1. Davies, Diane, 1948---Health. 2. Breast--Cancer--Patients--Biography. I. Title.
  RC280.B8D3615 2005
  362.196'99449'0092--dc22

                       2005016769

Contents

Acknowledgments

I give special thanks to my husband Butch and my daughter Krisi and my son-in-law Jeff, who stayed with me every step of the way, providing the love and support I so desperately needed.

Carolyn Salter shared long distance love and support from Australia through emails, cards, letters, and most especially, through her poetry. Carolyn lives near Walcha in the New England part of New South Wales, Australia, with her husband, David. Butch and I first met the Salters when they were here in the United States visiting some mutual friends. In December of 1996 we traveled with the same friends to Australia on a flying safari, of which one stop was at the home of David and Carolyn. We stayed with them for several days on their station where they raise beef cattle. They also ran an agricultural aviation company that was involved with crop dusting. In December of 1994 their son, Ben, was in an airplane accident that took his young life. Carolyn's first published book of poetry, *Once Upon a Shooting Star*, was written as her grief evolved after this accident. Her second volume of poems, *Hurdles Are For Jumping: Perceptions of Cancer*, was written in 2003 for the Walcha community "Relay for Life" cancer fundraising event. Having lost a brother and a mother to the dreaded disease, Carolyn joined a support group where she was inspired by the many people she met, young and old, facing a journey with and through cancer. She said the poetry just flowed.

The poems in this second volume were a great source of comfort and healing for me in my own journey. Many of them are reprinted here with Carolyn's permission. Her poetry also flowed for me when

I shared an early version of my manuscript of this book with her. She described flying with her husband in their Gypsy Moth, an antique open cockpit airplane. Their destination gave her six hours of uninterrupted time to let the creative process take hold. As she flew with the wind in her face and no communication available, she wrote these wonderful poems that captured my thoughts, desires, feelings and fears. These poems are all included here within the pages of my story. I thank Carolyn so very much for putting my thoughts into her beautiful and powerful poetry. Through all of her poetry, Carolyn hopes to touch the lives of others in "struggling with the kaleidoscope of challenges" in life today.

Several breast cancer survivors were instrumental in helping me walk through the days of decision making, anger and fear. I thank them for their many phone calls and loving support as well as their willingness to answer my many questions with candor, openness and understanding. Many thanks to my family and friends who were always there for me in so many different ways. Flowers and plants filled my living room. Others sent cards and still others brought food. Others made phone calls and sent emails and still others supported Butch and Krisi in ways I don't even know. Angels ministered to me through the music of Don Moen and his *God Will Make a Way* CD. The Breast Cancer Support Group in Hastings has been instrumental in providing answers and new friendships and hope. Others came and vacuumed, ironed, dusted and scrubbed. Some sent bracelets. Others drove me to my many appointments. Others sent gifts of books, chocolate, wine and comfy pajamas. The flow of love and strength and healing continued. Prayers were being said for me in my congregation of Cottage Grove United Church of Christ, at the United Theological Seminary and from coast to coast, as well as in Canada and Australia. Prayer and love lifted me and carried me through my journey *From There to Here*. I thank you again, my dear "earth angels," for whatever part you played in making that happen for me. I especially thank God for His steadfast love and healing.

Introduction

"The important things in life always happened by accident…You could worry yourself sick trying to be a better person, spend a thousand sleepless nights figuring out how to live clean and decent and honest, you could make a plan and bolt it in place, kneel by your bed every night and swear to God you'd stick to it, hell, you could go to church and promise properly. You could cross your heart seven times with your eyes tight shut, cut your thumb and squeeze it and pen solemn vows on a rock with your own blood then throw it in the river at the stroke of midnight. And then, out of the black beyond, like a hawk on a rat, some nameless catastrophe would swoop into your life and turn everything upside down and inside out forever" (*The Smoke Jumper* by Nicholas Evans, Delacorte Press).

My nameless catastrophe has a name—breast cancer. It too swooped into my life and turned everything upside down and inside out forever. You need to know from the beginning that my story, at this point in time, has a happy ending unlike many, many others that do not. My cancer is gone; no chemo or radiation was needed, just some radical surgery. I am very blessed and very grateful. It was not a walk in the park by any means. I know that my final chapter is not yet written. My hope is that the telling of my experiences may in some way help others along their journey through whatever nameless catastrophe they are called upon to face.

The pages that follow are my journal written in an effort to help me get my mind around the breast cancer journey that I was walking. I told family and friends many times that I knew where I was, and I knew where I wanted to be, and the only way I could see to get there was straight through the middle. The daily writing helped me to do just that. It helped me to get from there, a diagnosis of breast cancer, to here, cancer eliminated and silicone implants as a part of my body. It helped me to describe what was happening and what I was experiencing, and at the same time give voice to my feelings about those very things. To help make the reading easier for you, the events and descriptions are printed in regular font and *my thoughts and feelings are printed in italics.*

Many valuable life lessons have been the result of my journey *From There to Here.* As you read my journal, these lessons will be made clearer:

1. It is God's timetable, not mine. I've prayed for patience throughout my life. I thought teaching first grade was my ultimate lesson in patience, but then along came my husband's stroke and later my breast cancer. I wonder what other lessons in patience await me in my lifetime. My anxiety and worry does not and cannot change the timetable. It all happens in due time—in God's time, not mine.

2. Prayer works. It does make a difference and it can be felt.

3. Love comes to you in many different ways and forms. You just need to be open to it.

4. Life is good. The trees are greener and the sky bluer on this side of cancer.

5. Life is precious. It is too precious to waste and too short to worry over the little things along the way.

6. An attitude of gratitude is most appropriate and healthy. A natural outcome of gratitude is a desire to be of help to others.

7. Being a gracious receiver is just as important as being a generous giver.

8. Sometimes I do have to listen to what other people tell me. I do not have all the answers even if I would like to think that I do. It is an issue of trust and dependence.

Part One

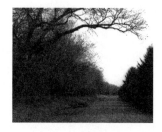

Diagnosis

I THOUGHT I KNEW LIFE
By Carolyn Salter

I thought I knew life
Touched all the facets
Shone in the sparkle
Plumbed the depths
Clambered back to sparkle
I have known life
Learnt from experience
So why now, this
This huge challenge
Life threatening?
Did I need to look again?
Perhaps
Could I make a difference?
Perhaps
I thought I knew life
But I am learning to know it
All over again.

I had my last mammogram in October of 2003. They called me back for a follow-up mammogram two days later, October 16. Some areas of calcification were seen on my right breast. They told me that they would like to do another mammogram in six months to reassess those two areas. I set up the appointment for April 19, 2004, and put it out of my mind. Here it is April 19. How time flies when you are trying to forget! I really hadn't given the whole thing a lot of thought until just a couple of weeks ago. I noticed in the mirror that my right nipple seemed to be about an inch lower than my left and that the right breast appeared somewhat larger. Then I remembered my mother telling me after her mastectomy in the early '70s, that she had watched her breast grow and change for over a year before she gave in and went to the doctor. I pretty much froze with the realization and terror of what I was now seeing on my own body.

Now my brain went into the "what if" mode. What if it was cancer? What if I needed to have a mastectomy? What if it was too late to do anything for me? What if I died? At least I hadn't waited and watched for a year. At least I was on my way to have the necessary tests. How will I ever be able to handle what lies ahead? How will my family get along without me? I don't want another woman to watch my grandchildren grow up and call her Grandma. I want to be around to see those grandchildren born, to see Krisi, my daughter, as a mother, to enjoy with Butch, my husband, our life well into old age. This is not fair. My dad died of cancer at age fifty. Well at least I'm fifty-six. I made it a few more years than he did! How do I learn to accept and live with this? Why me? Why now? I feel like the only person in the world with this challenge to face. Am I being selfish? I need to slow down and take this one step at a time. That is not easy for me.

This morning has found me strangely calm as if I already knew what was coming. I drove to Stillwater listening to my Rod Stewart CD. I found I was driving slower and slower as I neared the hospital—afraid to go ahead and knowing it was too late not to. As it was, I arrived a few minutes before my scheduled appointment. The woman ahead of me was late. When she arrived, they took her first for a normal screening.

The machine needed to be changed somewhat for me as they needed to do a magnification type of screening. The technician, as I learned later, had not done the type of screening I needed before on their new equipment. She naturally wanted to get the other woman out of the way before she changed things for me. That was perfectly understandable, but it dragged out the agony. The pictures were taken and I was told to have a seat, the doctor would be in shortly.

It was probably ten minutes or so before he came in. I have no idea what his name was even though I'm sure he told me. He put the film on the viewer and pointed out the areas of concern. I guess I pretty much removed myself once I heard 20 percent chance of cancer. I heard myself say that my mother had breast cancer and that I didn't want to wait any longer. He explained a couple of options for a biopsy, but I had no idea what he was saying. I must have agreed to something, however, as he said, "That's fine. We'll get it set up." He then told me that on a scale of one to five, one being benign and five being malignant, that I was about a three. *I'm no math whiz but I think the odds just changed. It must have had something to do with my mother's cancer.* He told me to contact my doctor later in the day, as he would let her know within the hour what was happening.

He left and the technician asked me if I was okay. I have no idea how I replied. She said that I had been a real trooper and had cooperated with her so well that she was able to get the pictures needed on the first try. She assured me that things would all work out—could she help me in any way? I didn't even know what to ask at that point. I think I was in shock or something. My world was going out of control and I couldn't do anything but go with it.

I was a little upset with the technician for trying to assure me that everything would be okay. If everything was okay, why was I going for a biopsy? How could everything be okay if I have breast cancer? I know she was just trying to be helpful. I need to be alone to work through things. I've always been that way. I think I need to be alone now for a while. Being angry at the technician wasn't going to help anything or change anything. So where do I put my anger? Who do I blame?

I got dressed and headed back into the real world. On my way home, I stopped at Target to pick up my Prempro. The clinic had already called but left no message. I, of course, called Butch immediately to give him the news. He was pretty silent. "I don't know what to say, Diane." He was not surprised either. I guess it had kind of been an unspoken thing that we both knew for a while but didn't want to give voice to. That makes it too real.

I called the clinic as instructed and left a message for my doctor. Her office returned my call shortly with the appointment for the biopsy set for April 22 at 10:30 A.M. I had a ton of questions between tears, none of which the nurse could answer. She told me that I had to call the hospital to preregister and that I should be sure and ask my questions at that time. Following directions like a robot, I called the hospital. I gave them the necessary information and did quite well, even if I do say so myself. I only had to look up my social security number, which I know like the back of my hand. Oh well. I began to ask my questions again and was told that she really didn't know the answers but would transfer me to the breast center where they could be of help. I declined as I was beginning to lose it emotionally. I told her that was fine—I'll just be surprised on Thursday.

I made a few tearful phone calls and then decided to get busy so as not to think. I used the power washer on the deck furniture and then turned it on the mold on the cement on the deck on top of the garage. Before I knew it, it was 4:00 P.M. and Butch came home. He let me cry for a bit. I can only imagine how hard it was for him. The big macho man with a heart made of marshmallow. We just sat for a while, together. I told him that I couldn't believe how poorly I was handling this. He reassured me that I had every right to be upset and scared—after all it was my body. *It feels so strange to be talking about it, the cancer I mean, in that way. That it's my body. It seems so unreal—like a bad dream but I don't wake up.*

15

Butch called Krisi for me and told her that I couldn't talk right then but would try and call later. The words were not coming, only the tears. Maybe later I'll be able to hold it together better and give her a call. Butch forgot to pick up his prescription so he ran into Hastings to do that and bring dinner home. I finished up the deck while he was gone. I did talk to Krisi a little later, through her tears and mine. We just spent a quiet evening watching TV and I crocheted. I was exhausted physically and emotionally.

My family knows about the upcoming biopsy. Wow! It's really happening and it's happening to me. I feel as if I'm in a nightmare and need to wake up and have it all go away. I don't think that's going to happen. I want my life back without the threat and fear of cancer.

April 20

I actually slept pretty well. I was exhausted. I woke up for the first time about 5:30 A.M. That's good for me even on a good day. I started the day with Butch's arms around me in bed and had a good cry. The rest of the day went by pretty well. I visited a student teacher. (I work part-time for the University of Wisconsin River Falls in their teacher education department where I supervise student teachers in their field experience placements.) I then came home and washed the big windows in the front of the house. Sunday we had had a lot of wind with a lot of dust, so outside furniture, end tables, and so on needed more than dusting. So I washed them all with soapy water and dried them with a soft towel. They actually look pretty good now. Butch came home early instead of going to the seaplane base for his night out with the guys, which is his usual routine. I made a quick supper then went to Bible Study. I came home feeling pretty good and went to bed. Waking up at 2:30 A.M., I couldn't get back to sleep and started thinking, which is not good. Butch woke up and held me for a while as I cried. He started to make love to me by caressing my breast, which only made me cry all the harder. I'm not sure if he was trying to comfort me, provide the healing touch, say good-bye to my breast, or help me say good-bye to my breast. The answer is probably all of the above. We finally both fell back to sleep.

I have cried so many tears that I cannot believe there is any more left in me. Butch is being here for me and I appreciate that so much. I don't even know what I want him to do or say. I'm just so glad that he is here.

I had an appointment with Nancy—my friend, neighbor and hairdresser—this morning at 6:45 A.M. for a perm, which I needed badly. I started this journal when I got home as a way to help me deal with whatever is ahead. I drove into Hastings for a few groceries and to get my watchband fixed. Working in the garden helped pass most of the afternoon. I moved hostas from down below to the bed on the west side of the garage. That was a real workout with the shovel and wheelbarrow. The harder I work, the more I'll be able to sleep—that's my plan. I talked to Faye, my friend as well as my brother's wife, for a while this afternoon on the telephone. I then went up to the farm and worked in my garden. Bob and Bub, friends of ours, along with Butch, cut some brush and had hotdogs at the shop over the bonfire they created. I talked to Krisi for a while and cried again.

This waiting is getting to be way too long. I wish tomorrow was over and I knew what I was facing. I think I'll take a Tylenol PM before I go to bed tonight. I already have a headache from crying. I know where I'm at and where I want to be and the only way to get there is straight through this thing, whatever it is. And that is the hard part—not knowing what I am facing. The biopsy tomorrow is the next step in this journey I'm taking. I wish now that I would have asked more questions. At the time, they didn't come. I couldn't get beyond the word CANCER. As my mind settles around this, the questions materialize. I have made a resolve not to hold anything back and to ask for what I need, both here at home and at the hospital. If I don't tell people what it is I need, I can't expect them to read my mind and respond to me. That will not be easy as that is not a part of who I am. I do need to practice that and I will. I keep looking at the clock and wishing it was twenty-four hours later.

This feels like "Judgment Day." The sun is shining brightly and spring continues to come, in spite of the turmoil inside me. I took a long shower, letting the healing water calm my nerves. Butch left early to visit the gravel pit in Hastings with a promise that he would be back by 9:00 A.M. or earlier. My appointment is at 10:00 A.M. at the hospital breast care center. It's only 7:00 A.M. This will be a long morning. Checking my email I read the *Daily Guidepost Devotional* for the day. As in so many times in the past, the reading appeared to be there just for me:

"Therefore, since we are surrounded by such a huge crowd of witnesses to the life of faith, let us strip off every weight that slows us down, especially the sin that so easily hinders our progress. And let us run with endurance the race that God has set before us. We do this by keeping our eyes on Jesus, on whom our faith depends from start to finish. He was willing to die a shameful death on the cross because of the joy he knew would be his afterward. Now he is seated in the place of highest honor beside God's throne in heaven" (Hebrews 12:1-2).

Paul wrote, "Forgetting the past and looking forward to what lies ahead, I strain to reach the end of the race and receive the prize for which God, through Christ Jesus, is calling us up to heaven" (Philippians 3:13-14.

The author of the devotional, Steve Biggers (Oklahoma), talked about running by a lake near his home. He described one long stretch where he had to run close to the water's edge. When the cold wind blew across the lake, this part of the run became the hardest. This is where he wanted to stop and lie down. But he has learned if he keeps moving he is eventually out of the way of the cold wind. He then goes on to relate this to his Christian faith by recounting times in his life, tough times, when painful experiences weakened his resolve. As he matured in his faith, he realized that God was always with him, during both the happy times when the running was easy and the cold windy stretch when the running was more difficult. His sense of God's presence in his life was renewed when he persevered.

Coincidence? Or God at work in my life? A strange calmness came over me. Butch came home earlier than I'd expected and the time passed. We finally got in the truck and headed for the hospital. We found the breast care center and I filled out some paperwork. The receptionist answered my first question by informing me that the results would be available in forty-eight hours, but since today was Thursday, I would have the results from my doctor sometime on Monday. That was not what I wanted to hear. *I felt like I had been kicked in the stomach.* They put us in a darkened room and showed us a video regarding breast cancer and the procedure I was about to have. It listed a number of high risk factors of which I swear I had all but one or two. (That was real comforting.) When it ended, I looked over at Butch who has this wonderful gift of relaxation. His eyes were shut and he appeared to be sleeping. I felt as Jesus must have felt in the Garden of Gethsemane. He immediately got my sharp elbow in his side and elbowed me back with a grin. "I'm awake!"

Catherine, my technician for the procedure, came in for me and said they were ready. I think it's called a mamotome. (Why do I keep spacing this stuff?) She told Butch it would be about two and half hours and told him to have a seat in the lobby. I knew that wouldn't work. He'd be off keeping himself busy to pass the time. I didn't blame him. I wished I could just leave my body there for the procedure and join him in however he was going to pass the time.

We started off with another mammogram as they wanted their own pictures, not the ones from the clinic. Catherine made the mistake of asking me if I had slept last night. The cold wind started blowing and the flood came. All of the tears that I thought I had cried came back again and I dissolved into a puddle. She moved me into the "core" room where the procedure would take place and called for a patient advocate, who came almost immediately to comfort me and assure me that I was reacting very normally. She told me it was okay to be scared and concerned. She related that 80% of the procedures done here come back benign, and for the other 20% they have options and methods of dealing with the disease that have pretty wonderful outcomes. I really felt sorry for the two girls. They were trying so hard to comfort me. They continually rubbed my arms and shoulders in compassion. I was on the cold wind side of the lake and knew that the only way to get back into the calm was to persevere and keep moving. No stopping here. I had my moment of self-pity; now it was time to move on.

The radiologist came in and Catherine introduced him to me. He never shook my hand or made eye contact with me, which I thought was rather strange. Perhaps my red swollen eyes were too much for him to handle. He did talk somewhat to me during the procedure but it was very obvious that patient communication was the job of Catherine. Believe it or not, I was basically pretty quiet and only spoke when asked a question. That is not normal behavior for me.

Catherine asked me if I was ready to start. I had to lie on a table on my stomach with my left arm up beside my head and my right arm tucked beside my right side. My head was turned toward my left arm and my right breast hung through a round hole in the table. The table was like a hoist in a mechanic's garage that lifts the car so it can be worked on from underneath, only I was the car and my breast was what was to be worked on from underneath. As in a mammogram, the breast is compressed in a vice-like device to make sure it does not move. Believe me, there was no way that I was about to move. The most uncomfortable part was the stiffness that began to set in after being in one position for a long period of time. Two biopsies were to be done on the two areas of my breast that were questionable. I did get to roll over and rest between procedures, which helped with the stiffness. I did an awful lot of praying as I lay there listening to the soft music playing in the background. I said the Lord's Prayer, Psalm 23, and any other prayers and verses I knew by heart. Some of them I repeated over and over again. I felt very little during the procedure. They used lidocaine to numb the breast, but being under all that compression for a period of time had to help with the numbing process as well. The only sensation I had was of a little tugging

21

and pulling accompanied by the noises of the machine at work. When they finished, I had a little difficulty trying to move. The nurse told me to roll over and I said, "Oh yea, right! I'm trying. Give me a little time to get this body moving."

Catherine was much more relaxed now that the procedure was over, as I'm sure I was. We needed to take two more mammogram pictures before I was ready to leave. In the process, my breast started to bleed again and few drops of blood landed on my light-colored pants. Catherine smiled and joked and laughed with me as she bandaged and bound my breasts for support and tried to clean the blood out of my pants. She told me that my core samples were there on the counter if I wanted to take a look. Two round dishes held four samples each of my breast tissue. I remembered the old potato guns that used a small round core of real potato as ammunition. That is what the samples looked like to me. They were about an inch and a half long and an eighth of an inch in diameter. So there I was, a sample in a dish in the hands of the lab and God.

Catherine teased Butch about taking me out for lunch and not letting me do any work or heavy lifting. He of course asked for how long and she replied that at least three weeks would work. She then laughed and told him that at least the rest of the day would be fine. She wished us good luck, as did the receptionist, and we walked outside into the warm sunshine of a beautiful day. The cold wind I'd been feeling was gone now, but I knew it would find me again as the waiting for Monday began. This was only Thursday afternoon.

I slept most of the afternoon until Krisi came for a tearful visit. She was upset about all of the waiting that I was required to do. We talked for a long time and held hands and cried. I know it made me feel better. Jeff, my son-in-law, brought pizza for dinner. So went the evening. Tylenol PM helped me sleep through the night.

I'm glad that this day is over with and I hope it never has to be repeated.

THE STARTING LINE
By Carolyn Salter

So here we are
At the starting line
Lining up
To jump the hurdles
Not our choice
Not even our sport
In some cases
But hurdles we are jumping
So bring on the starting gun
Let's get a run at them
Let's go over them.
Some we will not clear
But we will knock them down
And we will reach
The end
Proudly.
We will jump the hurdles
And our families
And our friends
Will cheer us on
All the way
To the finish line.

I could remove the ace bandage this morning and the other wrappings, but I needed to leave the two strips that actually covered the incision spots for three to five days or until they fell off. The tape holding the gauze in place tore off a layer of skin as I pulled it away. That burned a bit but I survived. That in fact hurts more than the biopsy area and will take a little time to heal.

Butch was flying the Super Cub up to Tower, Minnesota, today to deliver a part for our Cessna 185. He had asked me to go with him. We planned to leave the Cub for a few repairs and fly home the 185. It was a good trip. The Cub was tossed around a bit by the wind the farther north we traveled. Some of the bumps were pretty jarring, but I held my arms tight around my breasts to keep them from bouncing too much. Jim and Brenda, friends of ours, were on their way up to their cabin on Lake Vermilion in their airplane and radioed that they would wait for us at the Tower Airport and we'd go for lunch. It was good for both Butch and I to talk with them about what we were facing and about how hard the waiting was proving to be. We then went to the fish hatchery and the ranger showed us around and explained the walleye spawning process and how they were helping nature to be more successful. It was pretty interesting to see the huge walleyes swimming in the pens. Butch never seems to catch any that size. It was also good to be busy and have something else other than myself to think about.

After we arrived home, we decided to stop in and visit with Rita and Joe, Butch's sister and her husband who live just up the hill from our house. They were about to have a bonfire and burn a little brush and a few hotdogs. It was a relaxing evening. And the waiting continues . . .

Talking with family and friends is proving to be most helpful for both of us. The more I share with others, the easier it is becoming for me to talk about the possibility of cancer. I won't be able to do this alone. I need the help of all, including God.

Another day of waiting . . . Krisi has school this weekend so she won't be around to spend time with me. She is working on her master's degree in education through St. Mary's. Butch called from the shop and had me come up to choose the lettering for our boat. Crystal, a friend and local artist, was there to start the painting and needed to know our style choice. I stopped at Rita's on the way home and we had a nice heart-to-heart discussion. We both cried and hugged and cried some more. Butch and I met Bub in Prescott for lunch. We shared our news. It really helps me to talk about it. I don't feel so alone. Butch needs to know that he has friends that are willing to listen as well.

Butch told me that in the night I had given him quite a start! He said that I just sat up and let out the most blood-curdling scream. The subconscious mind is a real mystery. I must have been dreaming something awful. I don't remember, but I do remember him holding me tight until I stopped crying and fell back to sleep. *He's taking the "in-sickness-and-in-health" vow very seriously. I'm so thankful for his love and care.*

Tomorrow is Grandma's eighty-fourth birthday, and if the weather cooperates we're planning a "burnout" with more hotdogs, beans, and such. Target was next on my list as we needed a gift for the party. And so went the afternoon.

While I was out doing errands, Karen C., another friend and member of my "Sisters In Spirit," dropped off a "Happy Thoughts" planter of pansies. I'm sorry I missed her visit. I will phone her this evening.

I'm finding that the busier I am the less time I have for thinking and the faster the time goes. It is comforting to have family and friends share their love with and for me.

Another day of waiting . . . I feel like the accused waiting for the jury to return with a verdict. The only difference is that I know the jury will be in on Monday.

Today is Grandma Beth's birthday and a family "burnout" is planned. Hopefully that will be enough distraction to shift my thinking to something else for a while.

Butch, Krisi, and Jeff, as well as Butch's sisters, were very supportive today. Jeff hugged me and said that if it is cancer the medical community now has many treatment options with wonderful results. I guess he thinks it is cancer as well as I do. I'm beginning to realize that this whole thing is extremely hard on Krisi and Butch as well. I guess cancer happens to the whole family, not just the patient. I had a few phone calls and some encouraging emails as well. It certainly helps me to have other people know what I'm facing. They can't take it away but they can give me their love and support so I don't feel so all alone. I hope I can sleep tonight. I'll take a Tylenol PM and hope for the best.

The day is here. My heart jumps every time the phone rings and its only 7:30 in the morning. I keep wishing the day away so I would know one way or the other. If it's malignant, let's get on with it and devise a plan. If it's benign, let me get on with my life. Right now I feel so on hold from everything. Nancy called and asked me what I had heard. I know what a tough call that was for her to make and I appreciate it so much. Krisi just called to tell me she was coming to spend the day with me. She had called a sub and was on her way. (She teaches seventh and eighth grade English at a middle school not too far away.) What a blessing. It will be nice to have some company and a hand to hold. Butch said he would try to be home by noon. I continue to pray. I do not feel abandoned.

It's now 4:45 P.M. and I still don't have any answers. I called the breast care center this morning and talked to Shelly, the receptionist. She told me to call back at 12:30 P.M. as it usually takes until noon for pathology to get their reports out. I also called my doctor's office and left a voice mail message asking her to call me as soon as she had any information. I related how difficult the waiting was again. Butch came home around noon and spent the afternoon with Krisi and I. About 1:30 P.M. Shelly from the breast care center called back to tell me that she had talked with pathology and that the test results would not be done until 5:00 or 5:30 P.M. today. They would then be faxed to the doctor's office. That probably means I will not hear until sometime tomorrow. She suggested I call the clinic again and inquire how that would be handled and when would I know. My doctor does not have office hours every day either so I called again relating the new information that I had. Again I left a voice mail. About 3:30 P.M. Krisi called the clinic and asked to talk to a real live person and again had to leave a voice mail. As of yet, I have heard nothing from the clinic. I've about given up for today. Krisi sobbed in my arms before she left. I sobbed right along with her.

This is so hard for me and yet I see Krisi suffering even more than I am. She keeps saying how ridiculous this whole waiting game is and how rude and uncaring the medical profession has been. We need to have an answer SOON, and yet it will come in its own good time. Thursday feels like a lifetime ago. I wonder if I'm overreacting to this whole ordeal. What if it is not cancerous? Then again, what if it is? I still do not feel abandoned. I have the love and support of my family and friends. God will give me His answer when He is ready, I guess.

WATCHING
By Carolyn Salter

Sometimes I think
It is harder to watch
Someone you love
Suffering
Than to be that person.
If it were me
I would know
How I felt.
I could deal with it
But I am resigned
To watching
From the sidelines
And hurting twice
Once for you
And once for me.
I wish I knew a way
Beyond that.
For it is agony
Watching you
Loving you
And unable to fix
The situation.

Have you ever just known something? It feels even like more than a premonition about something—you just know. As I walked up to the farm this morning, I was remembering when I was in ninth grade. I was up for carnival queen that winter and when I came out on the stage the night of the coronation, I "knew" that I was the winner. I don't mean in a haughty, proud, arrogant way. I mean I just knew. I had that same feeling last week when we walked into the breast care center for the biopsy. I just "knew" that my mass was malignant. I remember thinking how this was just the beginning of my walking into and through this trial that I was about to face. I asked God to give me the strength to face whatever was about to come my way.

The psalmist wrote, "Turn to me and have mercy on me, for I am alone and in deep distress. My problems go from bad to worse. Oh, save me from them all!" (Psalm 25:16-17).

This is the Daily Guideposts' *reading for today. Even though I still have not heard my results, I've decided that enough is enough. I'm choosing to live my life as the true gift it is and not obsess and continue to worry over whatever it is in my breast. I will know when I'm suppose to know and will handle it at that time. I've wasted too many days being overly concerned regarding this issue. It's hurting me and my family way too much, and it is time to move on.*

Last night at 5:45 P.M. Donna, my doctor's nurse, called from the clinic. She told me that the doctor had just gotten off of the phone with pathology and that they did not have the results. My doctor does not work on Tuesday but the doctor on call has been alerted and will call me as soon as the results are in. Donna was most sympathetic about the length of my wait. She touched on my preliminary reports, the mammogram, and said that things really looked pretty good. She related to me that if she could personally run and pick up the results she would, but they were not ready and we'd just have to wait, no matter how hard it was. *Bless her heart. I felt that she really did care.*

So here we are. It's Tuesday morning and my life must go on. I encouraged both Butch and Krisi to go to work. They listened to me and decided to do just that. I have more energy than I've had for the last week. The sun is shining and I want to get out in my gardens. The weeds are already getting ahead of me. I know that whatever the results bring, we will be able to handle the days ahead. I have the love and support of family and friends, and with God beside me I will make it. Perhaps this is my lesson—perhaps this is where I needed to arrive on my journey through this trial.

I called the clinic this morning and left word with the nurse of the doctor on call to be on the look out for the test results. At about 1:30 P.M. I called the breast care center and was told that the results had been faxed last night, but they were faxing them again at that very moment. I waited until a little before 4:00 P.M. I knew once again we were closing in on the end of the working day and I would need to wait once more overnight. Krisi came about that time and called the clinic to find out when my doctor would be in again. She was told the doctor works on Wednesday from 8:00 A.M. until 4:00 P.M. Krisi then called and made an appointment for me to see the doctor the next afternoon at 3:15 P.M. Krisi had to pick Jeff up at 4:30 P.M., so she was on her way. Butch had the real estate tax valuation meeting at the town hall, so he left also.

The phone rang about 4:45 P.M. and it was the doctor's assistant that was on call for my doctor. She asked me about the report that I was looking for—was it an old test result or what? I pretty much lost it at that point and began sobbing and hollering into the phone. I was not very professional, I'm afraid. I related the entire story again and she told me that they did not have the report. I explained that the hospital had told me the results had been faxed last night and then again at 1:30 P.M. today. She said that their fax machine must not have been working because they did not have the report. She promised me she'd call pathology and get to the bottom of it and then get back to me. In about a half hour, she called back to tell me they had the results and that I needed to come in to talk to my doctor tomorrow. She talked about changes in the tissue and precancerous cells and early stages. "So it says that it is malignant?" I asked. She replied, "No, I didn't say that." She explained that since the doctor on call didn't know me at all, that it would be better for me to come in and talk to my own doctor tomorrow. I told her that I had a 3:15 P.M. appointment already and she offered to try and find me an earlier appointment. She double booked me at 11:15 A.M. and reassured me that my doctor would discuss treatment options at that time. I thanked her and hung up.

It doesn't seem quite right that a person has to call and call and argue their way into finding out test results. I'm disappointed with my clinic and the hospital. I was not asking for special treatment, just sensitivity to my needs.

When Butch came home, I shared what had happened. We both cried for a bit. He told me that I needed to have a positive attitude and move forward. He's right. He made me go with him to pick up a few things and a pizza.

Butch is sensitive to my needs and holds me while I sleep, or try to sleep. It must be difficult to walk in his shoes as well. I appreciate his being there for me. I will try to recover my positive attitude. I'm scared to death of what lies ahead. If they wouldn't tell me over the phone, it is very obviously bad news, especially since they wanted to have me talk to my own doctor. I guess my world is stopping, but that doesn't mean that the rest of the world will stop as well. That's a bitter pill to swallow and not very positive.

GETTING THE NEWS
By Carolyn Salter

I watch my life
Like a slow motion movie
The actress
Mouthing fear
Disbelief
But this actress is me
Not acting.
I am separate
Yet still aware
This is me
Getting the news.
Looking aghast
Seeing the mirrored faces
Of those I love
Crumple
Surely this is not me
Invaded by cancer?
I am still as I was
As I am.
Then the two "mes" merge
Truth dawns
Life threatened
Life perhaps shorter
I might die
I must face it.
And in the knowledge
As the full force hits
I, too
Crumple

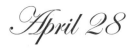

I woke up about 3:30 A.M. and couldn't get back to sleep. I finally got up about 4:00 A.M. and cleaned up my desk. I had a few bills to pay, flex dollars to apply for, and a ton of filing to keep me busy until Butch got up a little after 6:00 A.M. He left for Shakopee and will return to go with me to the doctor's office. We'll stop and pick up Krisi on the way. She continues to face this bravely. I know how difficult it is for her. I'm glad she has Jeff's shoulder to cry on. Our dog, Shady, and I went for a walk, which is good therapy and praying time. I then came back to my journal.

The telephone rang at about 10:15 A.M. It had been ringing all morning and I had been choosing not to answer. This one I picked up for some reason and it was my doctor. For a brief second or two I thought perhaps she was calling to tell me that the test results I had been given were not mine, a last glimmer of hope for a reprieve. No such luck! She started out by apologizing for her staff and the way things had been handled regarding my test results. She assured me that her unhappiness over this had been shared with the staff and that it would not happen to another patient. "I know that doesn't help you much," she continued to say. I did relay to her my disappointment in the handling of this matter with both the clinic and the hospital. She apologized again. She expressed a desire to meet with me at 11:15 A.M. as scheduled if I so desired, but that she was prepared to talk about the test results over the phone now, knowing how anxious I was becoming. She also explained that she had taken the liberty to set up an appointment for 2:15 P.M. this afternoon with a breast care specialist with the clinic. She explained that I did have breast cancer and that she'd try to answer my questions as best she could, but that the specialist would be better able to lay out my options for me this afternoon.

Butch came home about 10:30 A.M. thinking we were leaving for the clinic. We had a few hours to kill so we decided to deliver my car to the tire place in Hastings. We dropped it off and drove out to Apple Valley to pick up my new wheel. (I had hit a good-sized pothole this spring and had bent the wheel.) Then back to Hastings to drop the new wheel at the tire place so that they could mount the new tire on it. Well now it's noon. Butch suggested the Bier Stube for a burger. I told him that I was just not ready to face people and that I'd rather go home. I could tell that he wanted me to get out and about but I was just not ready. He complied with my wishes. We came home and made a sandwich and then left for the next part of this ordeal.

The breast specialist is a short little guy with a chuckle just under the surface ready to bubble over at any time. I felt pretty comfortable with him and Joanne, his nurse, pretty much from the beginning. My doctor told me he was a straight shooter and would cut to the point. She said he was honest, good, and a skilled surgeon. She advised me to ask any and all questions and that he would answer them straight on. Her assessment was correct. He did a double take when he came into the room and saw three of us sitting there. He asked if this was the whole family and chuckled about there being a dog that had to stay home. He was right. He very tenderly explained my situation to me, asking me questions along the way to make certain that I was comprehending what I was being told. He answered Butch's and Krisi's questions just as carefully. He drew diagrams to help us understand my condition and was very patient as Krisi took careful notes regarding our conversation.

He asked me many questions about my history; when did I start menstruating, how many children, my age when Krisi was born, when I reached menopause, family history of breast cancer, did I take birth control pills or HRT, and so on. When I told him that I was on Prempro, he told me to stop taking it immediately as the estrogen feeds the tumors. I told him that would be very difficult for me as I had tried to do just that less than a year ago. My hot flashes and night sweats returned with a vengeance and I slid into depression. I cannot go off of that without something else to help me through, I told him. I think he could see how agitated I was becoming over that whole issue. He just very calmly told me that I would be able to address that

34

issue at a later date and deal with it separately from the cancer. He went on to say that I had two separate areas of my right breast that both showed similar cancer. They were, however, not close enough together to take them out with a "golf ball." He then laid out the treatment options. First, they could try a lumpectomy, but because the two areas were not close enough together, this wasn't a realistic option. They would have to take too much in order to be successful. Second, they could perform a mastectomy of my right breast. And third, they could perform a mastectomy of my right breast along with reconstruction.

The lymph nodes on my right side would be evaluated during surgery. If they were not involved, reconstruction could take place at that time. If they were involved, radiation and chemo would happen first. The reconstruction would be done at a later date. The need for chemotherapy at this point was not projected, but the lymph nodes would tell the story. Tamoxifen (anti-estrogen) would be an option to help prevent cancer from coming to the other breast.

I had many questions about that other breast. The surgeon explained that of women who have had breast cancer in one breast, the likelihood of developing cancer in the other breast is 1% a year. Out of one hundred women that meet that criterion, one would develop breast cancer each year. He said if you are eighty years old, that's not too bad. But when you're fifty-six, it gives you something to be concerned about. I asked if it would be possible to have both breasts removed at the same time. We discussed the pros and cons of taking that kind of action. I explained about my mother having one breast removed and never being really happy wearing a prosthesis. It would slide around and made her feel out of balance. She had difficulty finding and wearing clothes that would hide that imbalance. The surgeon felt that I would probably experience that same sort of thing as I was not a small breasted woman. Reconstruction could be done, but it would be difficult to match up with my existing breast size and shape. After we discussed the issue more, he recommended that I have both breasts removed and reconstructive surgery done at the time if no complications with the lymph nodes occurred.

They set up an appointment with the plastic surgeon on May 4, 2004. He suggested that I raise my questions again on Tuesday with the plastic surgeon and get his opinion as well. After that appointment I needed to call Joanne, his assistant, with my decision so they could schedule the right amount of time needed for my surgery.

I asked the doctor if he would do me a favor while I was out from anesthesia during surgery. He grinned. I asked him if he would pierce my ears and put earrings in. He said, "You're kidding? You are not kidding!" He laughed and confessed that he had very little experience in piercing ears but if I'd mark where I wanted the holes, he would do it. I could tell by the look on Butch's face that we'd be discussing that one again as he is not a fan of any kind of piercing.

We left the clinic armed with books, pamphlets, and appointments. I now at least knew what I was facing and knew that I had some big decisions to make with the help of God, Butch and Krisi.

THE CANCER JOURNEY
By Carolyn Salter

We are on a third class train
Lurching menacingly to our destination
We know not where.
We chose neither the journey
Nor the means of travel
But we must go, nonetheless.
The journey is frightening
Many awful happenings along the way.

How will we regard the scenery?
With interest?
With horror?
With disbelief?
And what about the other travelers
And those who accompany them?

Will we help them if they have difficulties
On the train?
And what if their destination is not where
they want to go?
Can we help those left behind?
What will we learn?
Can we actually enjoy the trip?

We are on a third class train
Lurching to our destination
How we use this journey
Is up to each one of us.

When I was confirmed, my minister gave me this Bible verse: "God is our refuge and strength, a very present help in trouble" (Psalm 46:1). My fifteen-year-old brain couldn't get around that one at the time. I was a little insulted, feeling that he thought I was going to be in trouble a lot in my life. My fifty-six-year-old brain tells me that he was a very wise man. Every life has its troubles, and God is a wonderful place of refuge and strength, the One I want in my corner now and in all of life's other troubles as well.

Mastectomy—surgical removal of a breast. What an ugly word and what an ugly meaning. Cancer is another ugly word. How do I decide what to do? It all sounds so terrible. The end result of cancer untreated is eventual death. Mastectomy—surgical removal of a breast, an amputation of sorts—results in more life, more time to spend with Butch and Krisi and Jeff. More time to perhaps see grandbabies come and grow. More time to enjoy what we've worked for all of our lives. Do I really have a choice? Do I have one breast removed and then live in terror of the next mammogram, the next lump, the next cancer? Do I have them both taken and live with no breasts? What does reconstruction look and feel like? Do I really need breasts at this stage of the game? Would I be happy flat-chested? Would Butch

be happy with a flat-chested wife? I've never been happy with my
large size anyway. This seems like an awful way to get that changed.
Questions, decisions, decisions, questions. Life was easier before all
this came up. I wonder how much time I have to make my decisions.
How much time do I dare take to make my decisions before it's too
late? Is it too late already?

April 29   DAY 11

The following is the email I sent out to a few of my friends. It
was easier to put it together once and send it out.

Breast cancer, mastectomy, harsh words. They are even
harsher when you are talking about your own body. I'm working at getting my mind around all of this. I saw the breast
care specialist yesterday afternoon and we tentatively have
surgery scheduled for May 13, 2004. It will be at Lakeview
Hospital in Stillwater. If the lymph nodes are not involved,
I will have reconstructive surgery at the same time. We will
not know that until sometime during the surgery, so I won't
know it at all until afterwards. I have a 99-100% chance of
survival. Even so, I'm scared.

For those of you who like facts, I'll share this with you
from a book given to me yesterday titled *Ask the Doctor:*
Breast Cancer by Vincent Friedewald, M.D. and Aman U.
Buzdar, M.D. (Andrews and McMeel, 1997). This is what it
says about the type of cancer I have:

Ductal Carcinoma in Situ (DCIS) is breast cancer at its earliest stage. In situ is a Latin term meaning that the tumor is confined "in place." It is located entirely within the ducts and has not penetrated the duct walls to invade the surrounding breast tissue. But DCIS is cancerous. And it may spread widely through ducts, affecting a large area of the breast.

These tumors, also known as intraductal or noninvasive ductal carcinomas, usually are first found on mammograms as microcalcifications, *which are little specks or dots of calcium.* [That's what I had in October.] *They rarely form lumps and cannot easily be found on physical examination...DCIS accounts for about 10 percent of breast cancers.*

I have DCIS in two different areas of my right breast, which rules out a lumpectomy because it covers too big an area. That leaves me with a mastectomy. I really have no choice. If I do nothing, I will die of cancer and I'm not ready to do that just yet. I have way too much to live for and look forward to. So my enemy is DCIS and I have just begun to fight. Pray for the wisdom of the surgeons and that the lymph nodes are not involved. I'll keep you posted. Thank you all for your love and concern and prayers.

I talked to Obid, our pastor, today as I'm supposed to read the scriptures on Saturday at Carrie & Frank's wedding. Carrie is a longtime friend of Krisi. She is like my second daughter. I want to be there for the kids and do a good job. I figured the more people I could see in person before then the better I would be able to handle things. Saturday is not about me and I want to be able to support Carrie and Karen, my friend and mother of the bride, on that day. Obid said that he and Margo, his wife, would come over tonight at about 7:00 P.M. for a glass of wine and a good long talk and cry if necessary. Not to worry!

I did pretty well tonight with Margo & Obid. Butch was home also and I found it very comforting to talk about this whole ordeal with the three of them. We cried a few tears and laughed a few good laughs. We discussed my options and I felt very supported and loved. I told Obid that I would not be in church on Sunday and he assured me that he would pray for us "sinners" anyway, whether or not we were there. Then he just grinned. They left with a few tears and hugs and returned fifteen minutes later for Margo's purse. I guess I'm not the only one upset by this!

Sleeping through the night is tough for me. I can fall asleep pretty easily, but then I wake up at 1:30 A.M. or so and cannot get back to sleep. The night monster thoughts of the "what if . . . " variety keep me awake. I've started taking Tylenol P.M. so at least I make it until about 5 or 5:30 A.M. That helps tremendously.

It's real. I have breast cancer and I will be having a mastectomy. My emotions are on a rollercoaster ride. I feel like my life has been put in a box and someone is shaking that box as hard as they can. I continue to pray for strength to face what lies ahead of me.

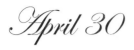

An email I wrote to my Gratitude Group this morning. (Gratitude is a small group ministry that I lead at Cottage Grove United Church of Christ. The group began by focusing on the abundance in our lives rather than the lack. This allowed us to experience the sense of fulfillment, which is gratitude at work. The natural outcome of gratitude is to share with others, so a ministry of outreach to our community began and continues to be our mission.)

I was just thinking this morning about a conversation we had at Gratitude the time before last about being a generous giver and a gracious receiver. Take a look at the *Daily Guidepost* for April 12, 2004, on page 110.

If I remember correctly, I said that being a gracious receiver was something that I had to work on. I guess I'll be getting my opportunity to practice just that. Thank you all for the card, thoughts and prayers. I would like to try and make our May 12 Gratitude meeting. I have a feeling I will need your strength, faith and love that day. I'll bring the Kleenexes. Love to you all.

The *Guideposts'* devotional was on Hosea 14:2 and receiving graciously. The author, Gail, had a neighbor who had helped her through crisis after crisis. She would send over little things like ginger ale when her family had the flu. She delivered holiday gifts and treats for herself and the children. Gail never felt as if she could ever return all the favors. It so happened that Gail and her family had to move out of state and the neighbor again showed up to help clean the house and pack the car. She brought a basket lunch for the drive as well. As the two women hugged for the last time, the neighbor burst into tears. Gail realized how much she meant to her neighbor. It suddenly dawned on her that by receiving graciously all the things her neighbor had done for her over the years that Gail had given her neighbor a gift as well, the gift of receiving graciously.

It was my realization that I too would need to learn to "receive graciously" in the months ahead. I've always been a giver. My mother, when she was still alive, would always tell me that I gave her too much or that I did too much for her. My reply was always that she should just learn to say thank you and let it be. I now need to learn that same lesson and practice what I have been preaching for so long. Lord, teach me to be a generous giver—and a gracious receiver. Amen

Tonight is Carrie & Frank's rehearsal dinner. I'm reading the scriptures and my hope is that I can keep it together. I've been asking for strength all day. One of the devotionals I read today was on Psalm 91. This psalm is the basis for the song "On Eagles Wings" which is sung at so many funerals and weddings. The song and the sight of an eagle always makes me feel secure and loved. The eagle symbolizes wisdom and strength, so I suppose that is why it is our national bird. There is something about seeing an eagle in flight that is so awe inspiring and reassuring, that "God is in His Heaven and all is right with the world." Living on the bank of the St. Croix River, keeping our seaplane on the Mississippi and having the privilege of owning a cabin on Rainy Lake in Ontario, Canada, we see and hear eagles daily. I've gotten so that I look for them as we taxi out on the water for takeoff as a sign that we will have a safe flight. I generally see one soaring overhead. It seems that if I don't remember to look for one, an eagle swoops into my line of view. I feel connected to the eagle in some way because of that. So today's devotional gave me a sense of peace.

I started thinking about that connectedness and remembered watching Walt Disney's movie *Brother Bear* with Butch the other day. As is now the case with many DVDs, much more is included than just the movie. There are outtakes, deleted scenes, and alternative endings to the stories. The *Brother Bear* DVD has games for the youngsters (or those that still think they are young) to play. Butch & I spent an hour or so after viewing the movie doing just that. One of the games included is called "Find Your Totem." Kenai, the main character, has arrived at a very special day in his life, the day the tribe Shaman is to reveal his totem. The totems are each represented by an animal of the forest. Your totem is the predictor of the path your life will take and what kind of an adult you are destined to be. One totem is the eagle, symbolizing wisdom and leadership. Another is the bear, representing love. You answer a series of questions and your totem is revealed to you. I thought I'd give it a try, thinking perhaps the eagle would be my given totem. I found that I was a bear and that love was my totem, just like Kenai in the story. Love is a good one to have. Without love, you have nothing. Love is what is helping me deal with this waiting time before surgery. That love is coming most importantly from family and friends. I know that my eagle is still there, however, a God keeping a loving eye on things. He will not let me down.

Rehearsal is at 6:00 p.m. for the wedding. I need to do this for Carrie and Karen. It was my turn to practice the readings. I started out with Matthew 5:1-12, the Beatitudes. I was doing fine until I heard my voice begin to waver. I choked back the tears and said I would try 1 Corinthians 13:1-13, the love verses. There was no way I could read any of this. So I politely said that I would read them tomorrow and sat down. Now I had Krisi and Karen in tears as well. This is exactly what I did not want to happen. The soloist reassured me, "Tomorrow, when the adrenaline is pumping, you'll be just fine." She of course had no idea of what I was facing. I just thanked her for her concern.

The rehearsal continued without any more scripture readings. Obid had everyone start over again for one last time. When it came time for the readings, he looked my way. I knew I had to do it tonight or there was no way I'd make it tomorrow. So I walked up there, took a deep breath and read both passages from start to finish without looking up or out at anyone. I gave a quick curtsy and sat down. Everyone applauded and off to the dinner at the Afton House we went. I can do it. I pray to God that I can do it.

May 1

Carrie and Frank's wedding day. My sister-in-law from Oshkosh, Wisconsin, Faye, is staying with her mother who is recovering from an illness. I spent an hour or so visiting with them this morning. Krisi and the girls had hair appointments and such and then pictures at 1:00 p.m. with the ceremony at 4:00 P.M. I planned to get there about 3:30 P.M. Jeff came and dressed at our home and went with Butch and me. I've never sweated getting up in front of a group as much as I did this time. I wanted this day to be about Carrie and Frank and not Diane; you know, the one with the cancer. I kept praying for strength to make it through and God was there for me. Not one tear was shed by this old girl and as Dee Dee, Carrie's older sister said, "Wow! You really know how to read!" I guess that comes from teaching elementary school for twenty-six years. I stayed pretty up through the reception as well. One tiny meltdown when I was holding Shannon's two-week-old baby. (Shannon is a high school friend of Krisi.) Margo and Sue, friends from church, stayed pretty much by my side and I found myself actually laughing and joking about what lies ahead. Butch tells me I've come a long way with this positive attitude stuff.

I hope he's right. I have a long way to go! I know where I am and where I want to be. I just have to follow the bumpy road that will take me there. With God's help and the help of family and friends, I will make it. I'm glad the wedding is over and that I was able to do the readings. Carrie is like my second daughter. She and Krisi were best friends all the way through school. I needed to be strong today for her. Mission accomplished.

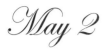

I had told Obid that I would not be in church today. I went up to the farm with Butch to have coffee with Grandma (Butch's mother). The poor dear is so confused. I told her about my upcoming surgery on Thursday and then her daughter Judy had surgery on Friday. She doesn't seem able to comprehend it all. Her world has become so very narrow as she ages. Everything she is revolves around her family, and that appears to her to be falling apart as we all age and have health problems of our own. In her eyes, we are kids and nothing should happen to us, ever.

I had intended to walk home but got busy in the garden instead. Before I knew it, it was almost noon and Krisi and Jeff came to go up to Afton Alps and help clean up after the wedding reception. Butch and I had offered our services as well. We returned by about 1:30 P.M. and I headed back to the garden to finish weeding and edging. Butch, Jeff, and Obid cut down two black walnut trees that were in the way. Obid wanted the black walnut for lumber. By about 4:00 P.M., I was pooped and so was Butch. We came home to shower and take a nap. I turned on the TV and watched a couple of movies on the satellite.

A character in the movie was in the hospital and they showed a close up of him in the bed. I looked at that bed and thought, That will be me in that bed before long. My mind started playing the "what if . . ." stuff again and I realized that I was scared to death.

Butch woke up and said he was going to shower and I asked him to just hold me for a while while I cried. Well, the dam broke, let me tell you. I was a sobbing mess. I realized that I did not want to die. I felt trapped by the whole situation, with no way out except right down the middle. Butch reassured me, "We can fix this, and we will. We will do this together," he kept telling me. And with no words left to say, he just held me.

I've come to hate my breasts for what they are doing to me and to us. The pain they are causing is almost unbearable. Butch is right, however. We will get through this together. I wish my breasts would just fall off and save me the agony of the surgery and recovery. Deep down I'm just a big chicken and a big baby afraid of a little pain. If I want to live, and I do, then my only choice is to face the agony and the pain. I don't know how I'll make it to the 13th.

We had many phone calls tonight. Butch very graciously answered them all and just said that I was having a difficult time at present and couldn't come to the phone.

What would I do without his love and care? What would I do without the concerned relatives and friends that keep calling, sending cards and emails of support? Love will get us through.

WHAT IS A LIFE WORTH?
By Carolyn Salter

What is a life worth?
A house? A car?
More adult toys?
More than this.
Education? Knowledge?
Much more than this
A family? Friends?
Oh. And more.
A life is worth love
As much love as can fit into it.
Love from all those around
And for them
Different love for each
And caring for all things
Knowing we are all
Little parts of the whole
Small sparks of the one great flame
All connected.
Complete empathy
All part of creation
And the creator
Knowing this—
This is what a life is worth
Love.

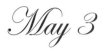

Again there were many calls, emails, and cards of encouragement and support. I don't know how people without friends get through this kind of stuff. I received a card today from Jason (my nephew) and Carie and their family. On the outside it said, "When your life is really hectic, sometimes it helps to stop and smell the roses." On the inside, "And sometimes it helps to stomp them into the ground just to blow off steam. Hang in there."

Wow! Is that appropriate! Next time I get really down like last night, I'll have to stomp a few roses into the ground. I love it! I'm sure in the next days I'll have opportunity to do a bit of stomping.

This afternoon I received a phone call from Carolyn H. She is the chair of the committee I've been assigned to work with at United Theological Seminary where I've just agreed to a three-year term on their board of trustees. I had sent her an email regarding my new health concern and what that might mean for me for the next few months. Rather than reply by email, she called. Carolyn is herself a breast cancer survivor. She had her surgery eight years ago this month. She told me of a time when she was on her way shopping before her surgery when a wave of anger hit her cold. She realized that she wanted to kill the person in the car in front of her. The anger was that strong and overwhelming. She turned the car around and headed home instead of into the parking lot. Surgery for her was about three weeks away, so she signed up for an intensive three-week class at the seminary. She went the first day and discovered after reading the first page of an eighty-page assignment several times that she could not focus. Her mind would not go around the written words on the page. She decided to drop the course and focus on survival. She told me that was my job for now—survival. That is where I needed to focus all of my attention, rather than worrying about the other stuff trying to crowd its way into my days. The letters of recommendation will get written for my students when I can focus again on their needs rather than my own. For now I have a big enough task, and that is to take care of me. Switch to survival mode and make it happen. She suggested a book entitled *Peace, Love and Healing* by Bernie Siegel. It gave her what she needed at the time of her cancer journey. I'll go online and order a copy for myself. God works in mysterious ways! I needed to hear Carolyn's message today and thank her dearly for it. I don't know Carolyn very well at this point, but I do believe we shall become friends. She told me that I sounded like I could handle this and asked if she could share my cancer story with the rest of the committee so they could pray for me at their next meeting. "Yes, please," was my reply. "How can I turn down the prayers of a seminary?"

Carolyn certainly is an "earth angel" sent by God to calm my fears. Her message that "survival" is my job and concern for the next few months seems to have set me free from the other responsibilities that I can not focus on anyway. I needed to be given that permission and she provided it for me. The rest of my life is on hold until I get through this cancer thing and that is okay! Now I just need to put that belief in to action. That is always the hard part, but I'm going to try.

I have my appointment with the plastic surgeon this morning at 11:45 A.M. I feel a bit like I'm going on a shopping trip, only this time I'll be choosing my new breasts! It is amazing how busy your brain can become between 5:00 and 6:00 A.M., between prayer and questions to ask the doctor and wondering about the surgery and thinking about the book given to me at the surgeon's office last week. *I'm not sure where one began and the other stopped. Perhaps it doesn't matter. Perhaps it is all prayer.*

I finally sat down and read the book on *Breast Cancer* by Friedewald & Buzdar yesterday afternoon. I'd been putting it off until after Carrie and Frank's wedding. I needed to focus on getting those scriptures read and not on me and my health issues. Now I can focus on me. As Carolyn told me yesterday, survival is now my job and my main focus. I need to be informed in order to ask the questions that will help me make a decision that I will need to live with the rest of my life.

The book was helpful. My surgeon had done an excellent job explaining things to me in understandable terms. The book pretty much backed up what he had said. Even though my cancer is in the early stages, because it is present in two different areas of my right breast the mastectomy is the recommended course of action. That is where I have no choice if I want to live. My left breast is not involved in the cancer, but being a woman who wears a size 40 D bra it does play into my decision. How will I look, how will I buy clothing with one big boob and one considerably smaller implant or reconstruction? What are the chances of the left breast developing cancer? And if that, then do I want to go through all of this again? The thought of facing just the mastectomy surgery blows my mind, let alone the surgery with reconstruction. What will the pain and recovery be like? Will I be this freak of nature when this is all said and done? Will Butch ever want to touch me again in a sexual way? If not, will that bother me? If so, will that bother me?

Everywhere I go I feel the staring eyes of family and friends. They seem to me to be looking at my breasts. I hate that! I imagine that will continue after the surgery and will be something I'm going to have to learn to live with. I've never enjoyed the stares or enjoyed putting my body on display. That is not a part of who I am.

I know that I am loved and supported by Butch and Krisi and Jeff and the rest of our family. And I know that I am loved and supported by many, many friends. Cards, emails and phone calls remind me of that daily. Some of Krisi's friends from work are participating in the "Race for the Cure" this Sunday and asked her if they could do so in my name. They will wear my name on their T-shirts and be there in my honor. (Hopefully Krisi & I can do the same for someone else in the future.) Butch tells me that people at work call him daily on my behalf. The students and staff at United Theological Seminary (UTS) are raising me up in prayer, as well as the members of our church, Cottage Grove United Church of Christ. Nancy, a friend in California, has her church and three other churches praying for me, and I know other friends who have done the same with their churches. Even Andy, a good friend from Rainy Lake, told Butch that he is not very good at praying but that he would try his damnedest. All of that is pretty much overwhelming and appreciated. How could one woman be so lucky to have that kind of support? God truly does work through community as my experience proves to me. I hope through all of this I never lose sight of that and continue to feel and appreciate its effects on me. I hope also to be able to provide that support for others.

Karen C. called this morning and left a voice mail message regarding lunch at the Levee and a massage and/or facial that she and Deedy would like to treat me to. Here is my e-mail response:

"I was on the phone earlier today, Karen, when you called. By the time I got done and called you back you were on your way to the sewing lady. Sorry I missed you. I very much want to have lunch with the two of you on the 12th. I don't think I could handle the Levee and I know for certain I could not handle a massage or a facial. Right now I'm pretty much angry at my body and I don't need any more people touching me. I hope that makes some sense to you. Perhaps later I would be able to handle that. I truly appreciate the thought, tenderness and love behind the offer. But it would only be another stressor for me at this time. Sorry. About lunch—let's save the Levee until later this summer when we can make it a celebration. For now I think I would rather have you two just here and bring a sub sandwich or something. As the 13th gets closer, I'm having a harder and harder time holding things together. I'm afraid I would be an embarrassing mess out in public at that time. I can be a mess with you at home and not feel so bad. I know you'll both understand. Thanks again for your love, thoughts and prayers. I love you both more than you know."

I talked to my dermatologist this morning. I changed my appointment with her from May 16 to May 6. I want her to check that basal cell carcinoma thing on my neck before we get into all this other stuff. I'm having a pretty hard time this morning keeping it all together. I cry at the drop of a hat. Please give me strength, Lord, to face this day. Colleen, a nephew's wife and friend, sent me a card reminding me to take it one day at a time. I'm trying!

My appointment was at 11:45 A.M. this morning with the plastic surgeon. We had the address and Map Qwest directions. Once we found the street we couldn't find the address. After a phone call to Stillwater Clinic with more directions given, we discovered the office building was connected to Woodwinds Hospital. The address really made no sense at all. We were just a few minutes late, which really didn't matter anyway.

After filling out some forms, we were led to a consultation room with a TV, couch, and two chairs. Kind of like a small living room. The nurse gave me a pamphlet on breast reconstruction, fumbled around a bit, gave me a look of pity and left the room.

I really did not want to be sitting there looking at pamphlet describing something that looked and sounded so awful. Gross was the only word that came to mind. I hated everything so far. The couch was hard, the carpet ugly, the people seemed cold and uncaring. I have breast cancer. I'm the one with a huge decision to make. This is happening to my body and I HATE IT. I hate everything that has to do with breast cancer. This is not where I want to be. It seemed like we waited quite a long time—I read the entire pamphlet and passed it to Butch to read before the doctor came in.

The doctor was dressed in a slick sport coat and tie and fancy shoes. He asked me some questions—the same things I had just written down earlier on their form. His gaze was not on my face or in my eyes but on my breasts. I felt like I wasn't really even a part of the equation—just another breast to build. I want this whole thing over and done with on May 13. I want to wake up with new breasts and get on with my life. I'm not very patient about things. I usually want something like this to be done yesterday as I don't have time for some reason to mess around. I'm angry and scared. Why is this happening to me?

My breast care specialist/surgeon had talked about a flap procedure where they take stomach area fat and muscle and build new breasts. If I did not need radiation, that surgery could be done at the same time as the mastectomy. It would mean a longer surgery, a longer recovery, but in the end a quicker result—a done deal faster. The plastic surgeon talked a little about that procedure but said it was very involved and would mean that I would not be able to sit up from a laying down position without rolling over on my side because I would no longer have the stomach muscles to make that happen. I would need to roll to my side and use those muscles to pull myself up for the rest of my life. *It was beginning to feel like I had no options at all.* He talked about the easier route, implants, and how they could start that procedure on May 13 by inserting the tissue expanders beneath my chest muscles on each side. The muscle and skin would need to expand to make a pocket for the implant. It would be the job of the tissue expanders to make that happen. The chest muscle would also protect the implant eventually and help hold it in place. This procedure would mean a number of visits to his office where they would fill the expanders with saline solution. I would come in once a week and have more solution put in, let the skin stretch, and come back the next week until I was as large as I wanted to be. Another surgery would take out the expanders and put in the actual implants filled with silicone or saline solution. Then new nipples would be constructed, and finally, the aureoles around the nipple would be tattooed.

It sounded to me like a long, drawn out process. Is it really worth all of that? I WANT THIS OVER WITH. The realities of all of this are finally starting to sink in. I have breast cancer, and whether I like it or not, if I want to live, I have to travel this road. I'm pretty much overwhelmed by all of this and have sunk into a major feeling-sorry- for- Diane mood. I want this all over, but now I have no plan of action that I want to take. I want out of this nightmare. It feels so unreal—this is not happening to me. It happens to other people out there—not to me! I feel so trapped, and the only way out is surgery to have my breasts and my cancer removed from my body.

DESPAIR
By Carolyn Salter

It's a long way down to despair
And I'm getting there
Too easy to fall
When the best way is up
They keep saying that.
But the ladder is high
And I've lost my footing.
Can't climb.
I need a rope from above
Pull me up, pull me up.
I fear I won't get there alone.

It's a long way down to despair
And I'm there.
Stuck there.
But I still see a fading light
Small chink of light

Up above.
Get a toehold, a handhold
Any hold. Hold on.
Hold on.
Keep my eyes on the light
It's not easy. It's hard work.
Keep focused.
Keep climbing.
Step by step.

Who needs a ladder
With my eyes on the light?
I can make it.
I will make it!
I've made it!
I've made it!

But it's a long way down to despair,
I know
I've been there.

We left the plastic surgeon's office with no decision made. I'm not sure that I ever want to go back. When the plastic surgeon left the consultation room, he told me that he would save the time for me on the 13th until later in the week. I should call his office with my decision by Thursday for sure, because if I didn't want the time someone else would. When he left, I said to Butch, "Well, he sure is a jackass!" Butch looked at me and said, "Oh really!?!" I got the feeling that perhaps he thought I was the jackass. *Everything feels so up in the air. I feel so helpless and hopeless about the whole thing. No plan, no direction. I just know that on May 13th I'm having my breasts removed.* I pretty much stomped out of the office behaving like a spoiled brat. Butch didn't say much all the way home. We stopped at Target to get my blood pressure medication. I cried from Woodbury to Cottage Grove to home. Butch just looked at me and said, "I don't know what to tell you, Diane. These are decisions you have to make for yourself." I asked him if he would have a problem if I decided to do no reconstruction. "Would you be upset being married to a freak of nature?" I asked. "Well Diane, I guess I don't look at it that way," he said. "I'd rather have you any way than not have you at all."

That really brought on the tears.

WHAT IS A BREAST?
By Carolyn Salter

What is a breast?
Small weight of flesh
A bump or larger
Yet these small bumps
Grew
Changing me
From child to woman.
They have been touched
In love and awe

They have grown fuller
Produced milk
To sustain new life
That dependent life
Touched in love and awe.

They have been a symbol of what I am
Who I am—
Woman
Wife
Mother.

Now I am to lose one
Maybe two breasts
A no breasted woman.

Is it possible to be the same
Without the symbol?
What is a breast?
Merely the symbol
Of who I am.
But not the real woman.
She lives within.
Not relying on a breast
Or even two
To define her.

Krisi and Jeff came for dinner. Krisi asked me to ride with her to
take some donations to the Stone Soup Thrift Store in Cottage Grove.
We talked about my narrowing options on the drive. She was most
loving and supportive as she helped me think through things. She was
able to point out to me a few things that I hadn't considered before. She
also helped me with decisions that were sort of already made but that
I needed to justify again to myself. For one thing, I had to determine
whether or not to have the left cancer-free breast taken as well as the
right cancerous one. I knew that I did not want to have one breast,
like my mom had to deal with the rest of her life. She had difficulty
dressing and always felt out of balance with one side bigger and fuller
than the other side that had the prosthesis. Clothes never seemed to
fit right for her. She did not have the option of reconstruction in the
early '70s. I shared with Krisi how I felt that everyone I talked with
now was looking at my breasts and not at my face. She is so wise. "It
will probably only get worse until this whole thing is over and behind
us," she said. "You know, Mom, you are so good about coming up
with some smart aleck remarks about things, I think that's how you
need to handle that feeling as well. You'll think of something to say

that will get people laughing and beyond the staring," she told me. "Use your humor to make it work for you."

Thinking through all of this with Krisi's encouragement, strength and love helped me tremendously. We had dinner and the kids went canoeing for a while. Butch and I walked down by the river to wait for them to return. They went into the old bar building where they have some stuff stored. Krisi loaded a few things into her truck and they left for home.

In spite of my family and their love and encouragement, I alone need to decide how to proceed with the rest of my life beyond breast cancer. How do I want to look dressed and undressed? What can I handle and what can't I handle? After asking God for His help with my decision, I took a couple Tylenol PM and went to bed. Thank God for Tylenol PM!

My family has been so desperately trying to help me, and yet they realize at the same time that I must make the decisions. If I were in their shoes, I think the following poem on the next page by Carolyn describes how I would feel.

I WOULD GIVE
By Carolyn Salter

I would give
My antique cupboard
With the marks
Of many generations.
The first magnolia
In a wintry garden;
The gurgle of
A special child's laughter;
I would give
My music;
Balmy nights
Under a star filled sky;
Love collected, cherished
Over a lifetime.
All this
I would give
And more
If it would take
The cancer
From you.

I slept surprisingly well. It must have been the Tylenol PM! I called my surgeon's nurse, along with a list of questions and a few confessions regarding my poor behavior yesterday at the plastic surgeon's office. She assured me that I was normal in my roller coaster ride of emotions and that health care professionals work every day with a large range of human responses and reactions. We again discussed the fact that if I needed to have radiation the reconstruction would need to wait until later. I tentatively told her that I would have both breasts taken and reconstruction started on the day of surgery if possible. *(Wow! That's not easy to say. God help me through this! My hands are shaking, along with my whole body.)* She told me to wait to call the plastic surgeon's office until she had a chance to talk again with the surgeon. Unlike others, she also told me that she would not be calling me back until after 2:00 P.M. or later that day and that I shouldn't wait by the phone for her call until after that time. That helped, as I have a lot of errands to run.

Alice, a neighbor and friend, called a little later in the morning. We talked for a very long time. God answers prayers in many ways, and Alice was his answer to my prayer for help. Two years ago Alice had breast cancer and opted to have both breasts removed. She also started reconstruction immediately. Her cancer was the lobular type, somewhat different than mine, but her surgery and procedure following was pretty much identical to what I was considering having done. She answered all of my questions very honestly and frankly. She told me I'd wake up from surgery feeling like I'd been run over by a truck. She had many lymph nodes taken, so her arms were involved as well. She also told me that the waiting now, before surgery, is the hardest part. After the surgery is over and you know the cancer is gone you are better able to deal with things. Before surgery, it's the fear of the unknown. After surgery, you know what you are facing and can move forward. She said she never regretted a day having both breasts taken, as the worry of reappearing breast cancer was gone. She also never regretted a day of having implants. When she undresses it feels good to her to still have something there. It is not such a constant reminder as a flat chest would be. The scars are fading and actually look pretty good. She even shared with me that she very rarely wears a bra unless they are going out in public and if she's wearing something shear. She has nipples reconstructed, but as of yet does not have the areola tattooing. She said she thinks she will do that yet, too. I asked her about the second surgery to remove the spacers and put in the actual implants. She told me that was just an hour and a half surgery with no hospital stay. Pain pills for a day and then Tylenol or Advil. Her nipples were also formed at that time. After the initial surgery, she told me I would need help at home. She pretty much sat in the lazy boy with her arms propped up on pillows for a few days. *Alice played a huge part in my acceptance of this all. I'm so grateful for her phone call and her willingness to share such personal details. I know I have a lot to face, but after having talked to Alice, I think I can do it, too.*

The surgeon's nurse called later in the afternoon to tell me that the surgeon believed I had less than a five percent chance of needing radiation. If I wanted to start reconstruction on the 13th, I could go ahead and schedule it. The lymph nodes will tell the final story. I told her to go ahead and schedule for a bilateral mastectomy (both breasts) with a sentinel node biopsy, and reconstruction started with tissue expanders if possible. I don't ever want to have to face this again.

I'm still terrified but at least the decision is made and the wheels are in motion. I made the call to the plastic surgeon's office. I apologized and moved forward. Now I need to work on that inner strength and positive attitude to get me through whatever lies ahead. I still dread the hours of this time before surgery. I especially dread Thursday morning and arriving at the hospital—kind of like a lamb to slaughter. However, I must remember that if I do not do this I will die. Once again I know where I'm at and where I want to be and the road I must travel in order to get there. I have a tremendous mountain to climb before I get home free—cancer free, that is! I have the love of Butch and Krisi and Jeff and so many other family and friends to help sustain me. I must learn now how to be a gracious receiver of that love, support, and strength. That is a life lesson that will also be difficult for me. I pray daily asking God to continue to walk with me and stay by my side. I know He will not fail me. I know churches in our area, as well as California and Australia who are praying for me, along with the whole community of United Theological Seminary (UTS) in New Brighton. With all that help, how can I fail? Even if I need radiation and chemo I should be able to handle it with that kind of support. I know Butch was relieved with my new, positively-growing attitude. I still have a long way to go.

My Sisters in Spirit (a group of women I work with and share a close relationship with) started arriving about 5:00 P.M. Vicki and Nancy came first, and then Freddie called from Ely. The two Karens arrived shortly thereafter and Nadine called. Lynn is still in Arizona but has been sending her love and support via email. We cried, hugged, talked, laughed, ate, and drank wine until about 10:00 P.M. I knew they all had to work in the morning, and most had a long drive ahead to get home. I also knew they were trying to stay until Butch came home. I assured them I was okay to leave alone and that Butch would be along shortly. He was probably waiting for them to leave before he came home to give us some privacy. He was out with his own support system—Bob and Bub. The "sisters" left me with a beautiful box of healing items, including Lady Godiva Chocolates, body lotion, wine and a special wine goblet just for me, Dan Moen's music CD, *God Will Make A Way*, and two special books. Quite a comfort theme of all the things I enjoy. The box itself was a beautiful gift. They know me well.

It really was a most helpful evening for me. I feel very loved and supported. I just continue to wish that May 13 was behind me. This is how a condemned person must feel while waiting for execution. Alice was right. The waiting is awful!

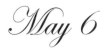 *May 6*

I'm feeling pretty confident about my decision so far. I'm still scared, but at least I'm down to one week and waiting. My plastic surgeon's assistant, Barbara, called this morning to find out if I wanted to meet with the doctor again before surgery. She was most helpful in calming my fears and dispersing my doubts. She assured me that I would be most happy with the results and that he did wonderful work. She answered my many questions and created in me a very different feeling about the plastic surgery ordeal than the feelings I had on Tuesday. I told her that I didn't think I needed to see the doctor again before surgery. She told me if I changed my mind I should not hesitate to call. He's only in on Tuesday at their clinic. I'm so glad she called. She had details that Joan, his nurse, couldn't help me with.

Later in the morning, Diane, a friend from Prescott, Wisconsin, called. Diane had the same surgery, removal of both breasts, in April of this year. *It's amazing how all of these people seem to be making their way into my life to lend their help and support. God at work in my life!* Diane shared her experience with me as well. She did not start reconstruction as she wanted to work this summer. She's scheduled to begin the process November 22, 2004. It was interesting to compare her more recent experiences with what Alice had to say. They were surprisingly similar.

When Carolyn from UTS called earlier in the week, she told me that my job for the next few months was survival; that is where I needed to focus all of my energy and attention. Alice and Diane agreed with her. Diane shared with me how ugly her chest was now about one month after surgery and that she was looking forward to reconstruction so she wouldn't have to look at it any more. She explained about the indentations from where her breasts had been but said she was glad they were both gone; she didn't have to deal with or worry about the returning cancer—at least not in her breasts. *I feel a real bond with these women.* Carole Helgerson has also called several times. As of yet, I have not talked with her, but Butch has. She is Butch's first cousin and was a close friend of his in high school. She was most helpful to him, and for that I am grateful. I will need to call her before the thirteenth. *My poor mom never had this kind of support, as far as I know. Her cancer occurred in the early '70s and was a pretty hush-hush thing at that time. It is important to talk and keep talking and to face the realities of what's ahead. I'm so grateful that I have those who have gone on this journey before so willing to share and help me along the way. My plastic surgeon's nurse said that I would be doing the same for other woman in the near future. I hope she's right.*

Butch and I flew up to Brainerd to Bill and Phyllis's cabin on Gull Lake for the weekend. The Seaplane Convention was at Cragun's, just across the lake from their place. Jim and Brenda were guests of the Bryan's as well. Wip and Linda, and Ed and Marilyn from Missouri, joined us for cocktails and dinner. Brenda told me that Wip had talked about having a going away party for my breasts. I reacted rather quickly and strongly that I wouldn't be able to handle that. Brenda assured me that she and Linda vetoed the idea and told Bob to back off. *I'm glad they did. Maybe later on I'll be able to handle that, but right now I'm a little raw. I'm glad we came. It's good for me to be busy and have my mind occupied with other thoughts. My upcoming ordeal sneaks in to my mind often enough. It's always just below the surface. Hard to forget about it when it's always there on your mind ready to take over your every thought. Next week is coming. Thanks be to God.*

Phyllis and Bill's newly remodeled cabin on Gull Lake is just beautiful. Jim and Brenda and Butch and I flew up in our separate airplanes. Bill & Phyllis had their Cessna 206 there as well. It was the annual seaplane convention at Cragun's. It was a good way to pass the weekend. For the most part I think I did pretty well. Friday night I had a hard time sleeping, so I opted to stay at the cabin on Saturday while the girls continued the second phase of shopping. It gave me time to sleep a little and think a lot. I did a lot of writing in my journal. What a perfect spot for that. I had nothing else that could distract me and I'm used to down time alone. I joined the group again about 3:30 P.M. for a glorious boat ride. Just like a scene out of the movie *Always*, we were chased in the boat by a water bomber heading to Cragun's for a demonstration. He dropped his load of water pretty much in front of our boat. We could almost touch the airplane as he flew overhead. What could be better? We had boats, airplanes, sunshine and caring friends! I had a bit of a meltdown when Neil and Eileen came to say good-bye and wish me well with my surgery at the happy hour before the banquet. *Talk about a way to clear the bar in a real hurry! Just start crying and they scatter. I didn't mean for that to happen, but what can I say? Tears and fears lie just below the surface. I'm surprised that it hadn't happened earlier!*

We flew home on Sunday afternoon, which was Mother's Day. Krisi and Jeff and Jeff's parents, Becky and Lowell, came down for a bonfire and a cookout. Krisi and Becky brought all of the fixings for the picnic, including homemade pie. Krisi and Jeff gave me a beautiful gold necklace. The pendant, in the shape of the breast cancer ribbon, had three diamonds. The card and gift were beautiful, and Krisi and I both cried. *I'm so glad that her friends at school are supporting her well. She had on a pink beaded breast cancer ribbon bracelet that she had been given by her aide. It sounds like her teaching partners pretty much check in regularly and give her love and support by asking about me and my progress. She has been so strong and helpful to me that I'm glad she can be renewed by others that care about her as well.*

The guys started the brush pile on fire and had it burning hotly when a storm came up. We had an inch and a quarter of rain and had to move the picnic indoors. The guys were soaked, having to stay out there until the fire was under control. The wind was doing some pretty squirrelly things before the downpour came. The storm certainly took my mind off of me for a while and that was good. Becky and Lowell must have brought the rain with them from Michigan. The last time we had a huge downpour was when Krisi and Jeff were married. That day we had four and a half inches as we tried to have an outdoor reception at the farm. The reception moved indoors, and a great time was had by all in spite of the rain. Today we cooked the brats on the Jenn Air inside, instead of over the open fire. It all tasted wonderful, especially since I didn't have to make any of it or do any of the work.

I hated to see the day end. I was beginning to get pretty nervous and uptight. Sunday night means the new week is just around the corner, and what a week it will be. I'd been waiting for the 13th to arrive, but now it terrified me. If I want to get on with life and over with cancer, I have to face whatever this week brings. The only way through this is to go straight through with head held high and eyes on the prize at the end. LIFE!

I had a hard time sleeping after about 1:30 A.M. I'm developing kind of a nervous stomach as well. I guess that can be expected. I got up and read from *Beyond Breast Cancer* for a while. It contains stories of hope and survival. I find myself in many of the stories. It's helpful to know that I'm not the only one experiencing things in this way. I did fall back to sleep until about 8:00 A.M. Carole, a good friend of mine, came to visit this morning with a bag full of goodies: caramel rolls, bean soup, homemade candy and rhubarb dessert. She went with me to Ptacek's to pick up a few groceries. It was good to talk to her. She is very supportive and loving.

This afternoon Butch and I drove into Hastings. I needed to get a cookbook in the mail for Marilyn Schmidt (from the seaplane convention) in Missouri and ship Amy and Eric's afghan off to California. I wanted that done before I went into the hospital so that neither would get forgotten. Then I mowed the grass around the house, transplanted some hostas, planted zinnias and sweet peas by the kitchen door, and pulled a few weeds. Gardening is good therapy for the mind and soul. Also, it's a good workout and should help me sleep.

The work of the summer season is beginning to play on me, and I have to realize that I just can not do it all. This summer is going to have to be, and look, a little different around here. The weeds will wait. I'm also fretting a bit about Memorial Weekend. I do so want to go to the lake with the group as planned. That, too, may not happen, depending on my recovery. I wonder how I will get my mind around making the list of the needed items to open the cabin for the summer. I just ran out of ketchup, of all things, here at home. How will I ever get my mind around all the stuff needed for the lake? With no grocery store close by to the cabin, I guess we'll get along with the stuff we remember to bring. I'm going to have to learn to let go of stuff like that and not worry about it. Seems like an impossible task to me at the moment. Why do I feel so responsible for all of that? I know I'll have the help needed. No one expects me to have everything ready except me! I've always handled it and will again in time. It's so hard to learn to be a gracious receiver when you've always been the willing giver. I'm working on it.

May 11 DAY 23

Alice called again today. What a dear. She had a couple of things to tell me. She asked me if the doctor had talked about saving my nipples to reuse. She had never heard of that before until a nurse friend of hers mentioned it. Of course it was too late for Alice, but she just wanted me to know in case I wanted to ask about it before surgery. She also explained to me how they will wrap my chest after surgery using a very wide and long ace bandage and how good that feels. *I guess she doesn't want me to have any surprises. She certainly has been a big help to me with the decision-making process. I hope someday that I'll be able to do the same for someone else.*

I received a note of encouragement today from Pat and Charlie, longtime friends of ours. Charlie just recently had his own run in with cancer. He's finished with treatment and back to work and I guess doing very well. "Hearing the word CANCER changes your whole life—you just look at things differently. The things that used to upset us are now just minor little things," the note read. *I'm beginning to understand that already. It is so very easy for me to let the dust build or the weeds grow and go for a walk instead. I hope I can learn to let go of some of my anxiety about that kind of stuff through this whole ordeal.*

Kate, the surgery coordinator, called at about 1:00 P.M. today. I was just about ready to call the number listed on the "Preparing For

Your Surgery" pamphlet when she called. My surgery is scheduled for noon on Thursday, May 13, 2004. I'm to arrive at the hospital at 10:30 A.M. She told me to take my blood pressure pill and the Prempro in the morning with just a little swallow of water. No food or water after midnight. Wear clothing that buttons or zips down the front and is comfortable. *Dah! The pajamas I bought, both pairs, are pullover! What was I thinking?* She asked me a bunch of questions and took down a lot of information, so I guess we're all set.

I had a pre-op physical with my regular doctor today at 3:15 P.M. On the way, we stopped at Herbergers to buy some pajamas that open in the front. I now have enough new pajamas to last me the rest of my life! The physical took about an hour and a half. I had to have blood drawn and an EKG and answer a bunch of questions—AGAIN! My blood pressure was a little high and my temperature was 99.1. I told them that I have been a little upset lately. The doctor wants me to go off the Prempro, as did the surgeon. I told him that I would need something to help me with the hot flashes and mood swings. We decided to give Paxil a try, as well as Vitamin E. He told me to wait and start that when I get home from the hospital. So that's the plan.

Vernelle, Butch's sister, called and asked if she could be at the hospital on Thursday. Butch was a little upset with that. We talked about letting people help in whatever way worked for them and us. We both cried for a while and continued to talk. I asked him not to get too crabby with people and to allow them to help. *He really seems to be having a hard time with this all tonight, for some reason. I guess maybe it's getting too close. Like I said before, it's too bad it wasn't yesterday and we were on to healing.*

Butch is really concerned about my comfort and level of pain. He plans to move the lazy boy from downstairs up into the living room in front of the new window overlooking the driveway for me. I agreed that would work and that I wanted to be on that floor, but that I wouldn't have a TV then. We decided to buy a new TV, which we could then take to the lake later on this summer when I don't need it at home anymore. *It's good to talk and to cry and I seem to be doing a lot of both. I feel bad for Butch and Krisi having to wait through surgery. I will not know what's happening, so perhaps they will have a tougher job than me.*

One more day! It's getting tough and I'm getting pretty nervous. I wish they could knock me out at home and deliver me to the hospital on Thursday morning. I have plans for most of the day tomorrow and Krisi and Jeff are coming for dinner tomorrow night. That will all help pass the day. I continue to get emails, cards, and phone calls of love and support. I do feel loved. I wish it was next week at this time! It will be in seven days—right? It's hard to not be wishing my life away.

I AM NOT ALONE
By Carolyn Salter

I watch the sun
Slanting rays
Fingers of light
Through the clouds
As if the fingers of God
Are touching me
Caressing me
With the knowledge
That I am not alone
All will be well
Whatever the outcome.
All I need
Is to remember
I am not alone.

May 12

I woke up at about 3:00 A.M. this morning and slept a little on and off since then. I'm feeling pretty anxious today. Last night and this morning people have been calling and wishing me well. I'm finding it hard to carry on a conversation. My mind is not concentrating and my ears are not listening to what people have to say. I guess you could say that my focus is elsewhere—where, I don't know, but it's not on chitchat. Everyone is so concerned and means well. I do appreciate all of the good wishes. I just find it hard to listen to them.

I have a busy day planned to help ease the tension. Gratitude Group will be here at 10:00 A.M. for our bi-monthly meeting. It will be good to focus on and learn about what an attitude of gratitude can do for us in our lives. Along with studying materials and the Bible together, we pray and support each other in our needs. Deedy and Karen are coming at 12:30 P.M. and bringing lunch. Krisi and Piper (their puppy) will be here after school and Jeff will join us for dinner. So will go the day. I still wish it were next week at this time. *My head talk is pretty much a constant prayer for strength and courage. I really couldn't ask for more love and support.*

PRAYER
By Carolyn Salter

Imagine prayers
Like little wisps
Of ethereal thread
Spiraling upward
Some catapulted by
Compulsive senders
Demanding, urging, arguing
Others pleading

Entreating
Others gentle
Beseeching
And others
Full of thanks.
Prayer threads
Coloured, glistening
Iridescent
Linking
Human to the Divine.

With all the prayers for me
I could weave a cover
Beautiful rug
To cover me,
Keep me warm
In the dark, cold times
When I am alone.
Yet not alone

For the beautiful threads
Of my friends' prayers
Shine for me
Warm me
Always.

Part Two

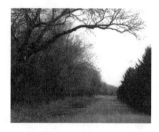

Surgeries & Healing

THE OPERATION
By Carolyn Salter

I smile calmly
Ignoring the rising terror
Inside
The surgeon's knife will be poised soon
Ready to remove
Parts of my femininity
My body
Never the same again.

A little fearful now
How will I react
Afterwards?
More importantly
How will others react?

Yet part of me is serene
What will be, will be.
I will take that
And work with it.
Changing negatives to positives
Helping others
On this same road.
Perhaps even inspiring
Hopefully inspiring

Yes, serene, calm
Yet, deep inside
Just now
For a small while
A little flutter of fear
For the unknown
Yet to be.

Thanks to Tylenol P.M. I did get some sleep last night. I actually woke up pretty calm, I thought. This is finally the day that I do so badly want behind me. Alice told me she remembers driving to the hospital with her family and saying, "This is so ludicrous. Here I am letting you take me to the hospital so that they can cut my chest up." I now know the feeling. It would have been better if Butch could have knocked me out before leaving the house. I'm sure that it was not easy for Krisi and Butch either. We left the house and drove to Krisi's. She would spend the day waiting with her dad. Jeff would come after work.

I survived the checking-in process. It was most difficult to say that I was there for a bilateral mastectomy. My name was called. Krisi didn't hear the nurse say that only one family member could accompany me right now, but as soon as they had me ready they would call for the other family member to come as well. She panicked and came to the door with tears in her eyes and told the nurse that she needed to give me a hug and wish me good luck before they could take me in. The nurse reassured her that she would call her to come and join us in just a few minutes and that she would have plenty of time for hugs before the surgery.

As I started the process of getting ready for surgery, I became terrified of what was to come. The sentinel lymph node biopsy had me just as terrified as the surgery itself. Would it be negative as the surgeon predicted, or would it be positive, meaning I would need radiation and chemotherapy and wouldn't be able to start reconstruction until a later date? So much was at stake.

Many people came in to help me get ready. I had to meet the anesthesiologist and his assistant and answer a number of questions for them. The nurse used a magic marker to put an X over my right breast. I told her that I was having both breasts taken. She excused herself and went to check on why my chart said one thing and I said another. When she came back in, she apologized and said she had misread the paperwork. Wouldn't that be great to wake up and realize they only did half of the surgery? I had to sign a number of forms, the IV was started, and I was given a plastic blanket that had warm air blowing through it to keep me warm. I was shivering, but I don't know if I was cold or scared. Probably both. The blanket did provide me some comfort, however.

My surgeon came in all dressed and ready to go. He asked me if they had given me anything to calm me down. He told me that I looked like a wire stretched so far that it was about ready to pop. I agreed that that was how I felt. They had told me earlier that I would walk into the operating room and would get up on the table with help. Then they would start putting me under. My surgeon said that they were going to change that procedure today for me. He felt that I needed something immediately to calm me down. "We'll get you in there and on the table without your help," he said.

My plastic surgeon was a little late in arriving, and the surgeon would not start his part until he arrived. The surgeon would take about two hours to remove my breasts. The plastic surgeon would take another two hours to start reconstruction by putting in the tissue expanders and closing up. My surgeon told the anesthesiologist to start by giving me a shot of something—through the IV, of course. I remember saying, "It's not working. I'm not going to sleep. It's not working." (My family told me later that just after I said, "It's not working," I asked them if they could see all of the beautiful flowers. Krisi asked me what kind of flowers I was seeing and I told her, "Why, pink azaleas. Can't you see them? They're all over the place!") Shortly after that I was wheeled into the operating room. I remember being moved on to the table, but I certainly don't remember much after that.

The next thing I knew I was in recovery with lots of tubes and monitors and lots of people asking me lots of questions. All I wanted to do was sleep and be left alone. Before too long I was being moved from recovery to my room in the "Women's Care Center" of the hospital. My family was there waiting for me. I remember hearing a lot of voices and trying to wake up, but I kept falling back to sleep. The news was good. The lymph nodes were clear, which meant no radiation, and the reconstruction process had been started. Obid and Margo, our pastor and his wife, were there. I remember hearing their voices and having someone wiggle my big toe. Krisi kissed me goodbye and went home with Jeff. I didn't realize what time it even was. All I wanted to do was sleep.

I do remember having to go to the bathroom. Two nurses came in to help me up and into the bathroom. It hurt like hell to get out of that bed and stand up. One nurse asked me if I thought I could make it to the bathroom. I replied, "I think I can." I remember her very gruffly saying, "That's not good enough. Either you can do it, or you can't. But we need to know." I answered back, "All right then, I can do it." I had no idea if I could or if I'd fall flat on my face. With a nurse hanging on to each side of me, we did make it across my room and into the bathroom. It was probably about five feet but felt like five miles to me. I couldn't use my arms much to help, but the nurse was there and did for me all that I could not do for myself. They must have been playing "good nurse/gruff nurse," and thankfully it was the good nurse in the bathroom with me. I know that bed felt awfully good to climb back into. Butch tried to reach over the bed rails to give me a kiss before he went home. He couldn't get down far enough and I couldn't rise up to meet him. I told him I'd take a rain check until tomorrow. He just smiled and squeezed my hand and left for the evening.

Two of Butch's sisters, Rita and Vernelle, spent the day at the hospital with Butch and Krisi. I never saw them, but it was a comfort to know that they were there pulling for me and helping Butch and Krisi pass the awful waiting time while I was in surgery. They did not come up to my room that I know of.

It seemed like a very busy night with someone in my room checking this and that most all night long. I drank a lot of water, which meant I had to use the bathroom as well. That was not a trip I enjoyed very much.

I certainly felt that I was in good hands. The doctors and nurses were most helpful and caring. Thank you, Lord, for bringing me to this place of healing. Thank you for the staff of this hospital and thank you for the advances in medical science that have played a role in removing my cancer and giving me another chance at life.

I HAD A DREAM MY LIFE WOULD BE
By Carolyn Salter

I had a dream my life would be
So far from this reality
Nowhere near this absurdity
Of tubes and pieces stuck in me.

Now the simple little things
Watching how a bird can sing
Feeling sun upon my back
Knowing there's grey
Not just white or black
Believing there must be a reason
Knowing we each have our season
Feeling mine may run its course
Knowing there is always worse
Loving more than words can say
Using each hour every day
Finding more, always learning
Living life, yet still yearning
For the long life I may miss
Yet grateful for it all, and this:

Cancer taught me such a lot
Cancer helped me find the plot.

But I had dreamed my life would be
Far from this reality.

DRIPS AND TUBES
By Carolyn Salter

Drips and tubes, tubes and drips
Taking little water sips
Lying here, told to rest
Lying here with no breasts.

Drips and tubes, tubes and drips
Lots of questions on my lips
Why me, why us, why this right now
Am I supposed to know somehow
What I should do, how to react?
And where's your plan?
What's the attack?
I'll do it when the pain subsides
I'll do whatever You decide.

Ah! Drips and tubes, tubes and drips
So many questions on my lips

JUMBLED THOUGHTS
By Carolyn Salter

Lying here
Unmoving
Sore from surgery
Can't soar just now
Grounded
Thoughts jumbled
No sense
Scents of hospital
All around
Confining
Constraining
Feeling like I've been kneaded
Into shape
Out of shape
Needed
Yes, I'm needed
By all those I love
Send my thoughts there
To be un-jumbled
So they can come back
Floating
Soaring
Settling back to me
Clear thoughts

Alice was right; I do feel like I've been run over by a truck. But the good news is that the lymph nodes were not involved with the cancer. The tumors were *in situ*, meaning they had not moved out of the ducts in my breast. I could stand the pain knowing that the cancer was gone from my body and that reconstruction had started as planned. I was a most happy camper.

The day passed rather quickly with doctors and nurses in and out and family and friends stopping by for short visits as to not tire me out. I even had phone calls from friends vacationing in Alaska and Wyoming. Flowers and gifts were delivered and love shared. I have never felt so loved and supported before by so many people in my life. Obid stopped by again, and we said prayers of thanks and healing. My journal writing today was hardly readable. I tried. I had four drain tubes, two under each arm, to help drain away the fluid that collects as a part of the healing process. They made it pretty difficult to use my arms for anything but just hanging there. Writing and wiping were most difficult.

By evening, I was beginning to feel pretty anxious. I was moving around better and adjusting to the drain tubes and the bandages, but an overwhelming sadness came over me in spite of all the love and support that was being sent my way. Sleep was very difficult and I found myself awake well into the morning hours. The nurse suggested I take something to make me sleep. When Krisi was born, I was given "something to make me sleep," and it had the opposite reaction in my body and charged me up instead. That was an awful experience that I did not want to repeat. The nurse explained to me that medications have changed so much in the last twenty-five years that that medication was probably no longer in use. She suggested I try what they had, as I really did need to get some rest. I finally agreed and was able to relax and sleep for a few hours.

Hospital time moves on no matter how much sleep you've had the night before. It suddenly dawned on me that I had not taken a Prempro since the morning of May 13. That was two days ago. Perhaps that was the cause of my anxiety. I talked it over with the nurse. She agreed with me that missing my Prempro would make me anxious. Hormone replacement does work in that way. She called my doctor and received permission to give me the Prempro. The morning passed rather quickly again between doctor visits; the nurse helped me wash my hair with "Hair," a rinse-free shampoo in a cap, and Butch came for a visit. In spite of my lack of sleep, I really felt pretty good.

The doctor told me that I could go home if I wanted to. I was ready, but a little concerned about the drain tubes and the pain pack that was installed. The pain pack was a bag of pain relief medication that fed directly into my incisions through a very tiny tube. I could control the amount that I wanted or needed. It was in a black bag with a strap over my shoulder. It didn't make moving any easier but certainly helped the pain. The pain pack was disconnected, which gave me a little more ease in movement—one less thing to worry about. Butch was trained in how to take care of the drain tubes. We were given pages of instructions and appointments, along with bags of bandages and what not to keep me comfortable. We carefully left for home. *Wow, what a beautiful day. I don't remember the weather outside—but inside the car it was warm and sunny. I had the surgery behind me. The cancer was gone and I was on my way home to healing and hopefully health. I had certainly climbed the large mountain that was in my path from there to here! But I did hurt, and I was pooped!*

I came home from the hospital early this afternoon with four drain tubes, hands full of pills to relieve the pain and stop infection, a box of rubber gloves for draining the tubes, bandages, ace wraps, even a product to dry wash my hair (my dirty hair is driving me nuts).

Rita and Joe, Butch's sister and husband, had carried the recliner up from the family room into the living room and placed it in front of my bay window overlooking the driveway. What a perfect spot for me to watch the goings and comings and to heal. I had Butch cover the chair with a quilt that my grandmother from one side had sewn the pattern together and my grandmother from the other side had put together with a backing and padding and then quilted for me. I felt in a sense wrapped in their love. I used bed pillows to prop up my arms and to keep handy in case I needed something to hug while I coughed or sneezed. Butch bought a new TV and wall mount for my healing corner. He plugged in a telephone within my reach and moved my CD player so that I could operate it with the remote control. I had my pills and water close at hand and a bathroom just a short walk done the hall. Talk about comfort and love! I was hurting, but it felt so wonderful to be home and on the healing side of things. Talk about being spoiled! I am so blessed.

The delivery trucks kept coming all afternoon. We joked about them having an accident running into each other in the driveway. By evening, my living room was filled with beautiful arrangements and lovely plants. We had brought a car full home with us from the hospital as well. I told Butch that it smelled like a funeral home in our living room. He just laughed and told me that it was much better than a funeral home. He said, "You are alive and here to enjoy the plants and flowers. That seems much better to me!" He was right and enjoy I did. I pretty much spent my time listening to Don Moen's music CD, *God Will Make A Way*, and sleeping and resting.

Butch became "Nurse Butch" as he cared for me ever so gently and lovingly. Every few hours he had to drain and measure and record the fluid collecting in all four of my drains. He cooked and brought me food, and made sure I had plenty of water and that I took my pills on time. He helped me wash up and settle into my chair for the evening. Krisi, of course, was at hand when Butch couldn't be there. She then took over the same duties.

It was the most comfortable for me in the recliner. The chair was a gift from my dad to Butch for his service many years ago when my mother had her mastectomy and needed to be taken daily for radiation treatments. Butch, being in business for himself at the time, had more flexibility in his schedule and was able to do that driving for her so my dad didn't have to take off from work quite so much. How ironic that I was now using that same chair to bring me comfort after my own surgery of the same kind.

Thank you, Lord, for seeing me through my surgery and for sending "earth angels" in the form of Butch, Krisi and family and friends to care for me. I am very blessed and so very grateful. Amen.

May 16

Each day I'm feeling better and stronger. I start out the night sleeping in our bed, then about 2:30 A.M. or so I move downstairs to my recliner. I still find the recliner to be most comfortable. It's easier to prop my arms up on the pillows when I'm half sitting up. We have a large security light that shines in the part of the lawn that I can see from my window. I do enjoy the view, even in the wee hours of the morning when sleep will not come.

My brother and his wife from Oshkosh, Wisconsin, Dave and Faye, have been here all weekend. Faye is an RN, so she has been relieving Butch of his nursing duties and helping me out a lot. It was good to have them here, but they are heading home this afternoon. More visits from family and friends helped to pass the day. Our friend, Andy, from up at the lake, came to visit, bringing gifts of homemade mushroom soup with sour cream, a bouquet of lily of the valley that he had picked for me, and a large trivet that he had made out of wine corks. He served me my soup right in my recliner and generally made me feel pretty special. The newlyweds, Carrie and Frank, even stopped in to wish me well. The telephone keeps ringing and best wishes keep pouring in. *I'm certainly not traveling this road alone by any means. What a blessing!*

Last night Vicki, one of my "Sisters in Spirit", brought dinner and helped me wash my hair again with that bed head stuff. How wonderful to have friends that I feel so comfortable with, and they with me that she can wash my hair and do such personal things for me. What a blessing to be sure.

After she left, I decided to try a bath. Butch wanted to know if I felt I needed some help. Of course I was sure I could do it myself. I ran about an inch of hot soapy water into the tub and carefully crawled in. It felt so wonderful! I just sat there for a few minutes enjoying the healing power of water. When I started to try to wash myself, I realized that it was too painful to move my arms in such a way as needed to scrub my body. I called for Butch and found that he was waiting right outside the bathroom door, knowing full well that I would not be successful in accomplishing my mission. He helped me out of the tub and had me sit on the edge. He gently and ever so carefully washed my back, neck and arms. "Did you ever think thirty some years ago when we got married that one day I'd be giving you a bath like this?" he laughed. I replied, "You mean me with this flat chest? I'm just glad that there is no hidden camera for Funniest Home Videos."

It felt rather strange to have Butch help me dry and dress and all, but it was wonderful to feel clean and ever so loved. It was one of the tenderest moments of our marriage. I'm working very hard on being a "gracious receiver." It's not easy. For some reason, I have a hard time letting Butch and Krisi wait on me. I feel so bad that they have to do that stuff for me. I also know how helpless they feel with this whole thing. By helping me in this way it makes them feel better, and so do I.

We came downstairs armed with shampoo and a towel. Butch carefully washed my hair in the kitchen sink. He was so gentle and caring and it felt sooooooo good. I hate dirty hair!

I told Beth, my mother-in-law, that she should be so proud of her son and his care for me. She cried, feeling as helpless as everyone else. She really didn't know how to react to the compliment. I guess she has a hard time being a gracious receiver as well as I do. I'm so glad to be on the healing side of surgery even if I am uncomfortable. A couple more days of drains should do it, I hope. Maybe by Thursday the last two will be pulled. The mailbox is loaded daily with cards and letters of encouragement. *I didn't realize that I was so loved! The prayers, cards, letters, and caring acts of kindness are certainly lifting me up and carrying me through this breast cancer journey. Thank God!*

Krisi came after school to "take care" of me. She changed the bedding, swept the floors, watered plants, folded clothes, shook rugs and who knows what all else. What a gift she has been all of her life, especially now. I was in the process of telling her it was time to go home and take care of her own husband when in he drove. They fixed brats on the grill for dinner. It was good for the four of us to have some quiet family time to discuss future options regarding our estate planning process.

OPPOSITES
By Carolyn Salter

The dark side of the earth
Will soon be the bright side
Happiness of being together
Follows the poignancy
Of being apart.
Ups and downs
Positives, negatives
All in balance
Needing each to appreciate
The other

I've been doing a lot of complaining about the drain tubes. Butch asked me what they felt like. I told him it was like taking a broom handle and putting it behind your back and then draping your arms up and over the front of it on each side. THEN, take two wooden pencils and shove them under your skin, leaving about two to three inches protruding. Now move, and lie down, and stand up, and pee and wipe. I think I drew a pretty good picture for him.

I was hurting pretty good before bed tonight. About all I could do was cry and swallow pills. I cleaned up as best I could with such limited use of my arms and then lay down on the bed that looked so inviting. I slept until the news came on and then decided to get up and go shut off the computer. It was pretty well locked up. I had been online earlier viewing some pictures of the wedding that Frank and Carrie emailed me, and Butch had tried to run a search that really took care of things. The date had even reset to January 1904! No way am I going back to that date! I'd much rather look ahead at this point. As the tears streamed down my face, I tried to type a command or two to get things straightened out. What a miserable mess! That is, both me and the computer. Butch helped me to get things shut down and then helped me to go to "chair" instead of bed. My lazy boy with a couple of pillows under each arm is the BEST! Two pain pills and I was set. I slept very hard for about four hours. Of course, by then I needed to use the bathroom, as well as let Shady, our dog, out and in. Two more pain pills and the next thing I knew it was 6:00 A.M. *Thank God!*

May 18   DAY 30

We had an appointment this morning with the plastic surgeon. He was able to take out two of the four drain tubes. Hurrah!!! I was a little nervous about that procedure and how much it would hurt. The doctor told me to lie down and take a deep breath. He asked me to take a second deep breath and pulled on the tube at the same time. Out it came. No problem. My concern was for nothing, as I really didn't feel a thing. My underarms, however, are very sore from the drain sites. I think that hurts more than the actual incisions. I must have been doing some complaining as he told me that I needed to learn to walk before I could run, and that it all takes time. That is just not part of my nature, but I guess that is another lesson I need to learn. He taped me somewhat differently, so hopefully my fat arms won't rub as much. It feels pretty tight, but maybe that is a good thing. Butch took me home and headed for work.

Later in the afternoon Butch called to check on me. I told him I was going to walk out to the mailbox at the end of our driveway. He told me no, that I had better stay close to my chair. "Remember, you have to walk before you can run." *That's a tough one for me. Having people wait on me is another tough one. Today when we left the doctor's office I had a hard time opening the door. My chest pulls when I do things like that. I had to step aside and let Butch open the door for me. I do feel today like someone has been stomping on my chest. I guess I'll just give in and be lazy. Perhaps lazy is the wrong word to use.*

89

ONE DAY AT A TIME
By Carolyn Salter

One step
Then another
Face it as it comes
Not before.
It may not come.

One step
Then another
Take each step
And live it
Love it
Use it
Fight the fight
Together
Live the love
Together
One step
Then another
One day at a time

I'm still pretty much in misery with my arms. Butch called the doctor's office and talked to the assistant, Barbara. She told us to come in to the office and she would pull the remaining two tubes. Oh, happy day!!!!

Barbara and I had visited by telephone before the surgery. She's the one I asked to apologize to the plastic surgeon for my poor attitude and behavior. We talked at length that day about how I felt when I first consulted with the doctor. Barbara is a very empathetic, caring individual. She made me feel so comfortable and normal regarding my fears and anger. She assured me that they deal daily with patients facing cancer and understand the anger. We also talked about the word CANCER and what that means, and how you feel when you first hear it used in connection with your own body. It is a terrifying experience. She did raise my concerns with the doctor, reminding him that each patient is hearing this stuff for the first time, not day in and day out as he does. She said that he told her that no one had ever said that to him before. *We all need reminders to be human now and again. As my outlook and attitude improve, so do my feelings regarding the plastic surgeon. He is treating me like a person, not just another breast to reconstruct. He smiles and teases somewhat and seems much more approachable. He was probably that way all along. It was my attitude that needed adjusting. I wanted to be anywhere but at the beginning of a breast cancer journey.*

Barbara again was very thorough today in removing the last two tubes. She helped me breathe through as she pulled them out. It stung a little, but I already feel better having them gone. She told me that I could shower in the morning! She asked Butch to stand by outside while I showered as people that are weak sometimes get a little light headed. He told her he'd have no problem just getting right in with me. In fact, he thought perhaps he'd even take the dog in and we'd all get clean at once. We told her about Butch giving me a bath the other night and how we ended up laughing about it being a funniest home video. "I don't think so!" she replied. "It sounds very tender to me."

I had related the same incident earlier to a friend of mine from the seminary when she called to check on me. She said surely not funniest home video, but a most tender loving moment. *I guess I'd have to agree. She said, "Your husband must love you very much." Again I have to agree. He has become quite a tender nurse. Who knew?*

Boy can I sleep! I load my Bose Music System with CDs, get comfy in my lazy boy, and sleep and heal. The reoccurring theme of a "slow and easy" recovery keeps coming back to me. Slow and easy does feel good. One card today read, "The path of healing is an ever changing journey, with threads of faith and courage softly intertwined among the gentle colors of hope." *I'm a believer. I'm so happy to be on this side of surgery. Tomorrow will be one week. I've come a long way and do plan to continue to rest and relax my way through this as much as possible.*

Tomorrow I see my original surgeon and Friday the oncologist. This has been a busy week, what with all of the doctor appointments and the sleeping!

When Krisi was here yesterday, she asked me if I remembered the flowers in the pre-op room. She said they'd given me something to relax and I kept saying, "It's not working. It's not working. I could get right up and walk out of here!" Then I asked them if they could see the beautiful flowers. I can just imagine the two of them grinning at each other over my head and snickering. Krisi said she asked me what kind of flowers they were, and I told her, "Why, pink azaleas!" Today when we got home from the doctor's office, what was waiting by the door but a huge, big beautiful pink azalea from some friends. Coincidence, or have they heard the story?

My arms are feeling much better for sure. It will be good to remove the tape from under them in the shower in the morning, if not before.

Friends have been showing up with dinner every night for us. What a thoughtful treat! It's great to have the food, but even more enjoyable is to have the friends stay and eat with us. Butch has made that rule: If you bring food, you must stay and enjoy it with us. It has been great.

May 20

We had an appointment early this morning with the surgeon who did the mastectomy. All went very well. The pathology report confirmed that my lymph nodes were clear. *GOOD NEWS!* The doctor felt that I would not need chemotherapy, but he wanted me to visit with an oncologist anyway. Then he winked and told me to try and stay away from him. He said he really didn't want to see me in his office again. He chuckled through a good-bye and good luck. I'm totally in the plastic surgeon's hands for the rest of my healing. We left the hospital and drove to Taylors Falls, Minnesota, to look at a tractor that Butch was interested in. I slept most of the way. It's great to have such a nice, comfortable car.

Another good friend, Linda, came this afternoon and did my ironing. Bless her heart. *I even let her! Bless my heart. I'm learning. That is a big step for me in acceptance of my circumstances.* Two more friends showed up later, Nadine and Karen, with dinner. Butch saw all of the women here and adjourned to the shop to work on something. It's good for him to have a break from his nursing duties. I talked the girls into staying and eating with me. It wasn't very hard to convince them to stay. I was pretty tired by the time everyone left. But it was a good tired, and a very good day!

This afternoon we met with an oncologist at Lakeview Hospital in Stillwater. He was most kind and personable. We must have been there for almost two hours. We talked about me and my family history with cancer. He explained that I have an eight percent chance of developing cancer somewhere else in my body in the next ten years. With chemotherapy, they could lower that to six percent. He felt that the side effects and risks of chemo, heart disease and leukemia, would be greater than the two percent increase in my chances of not developing more cancer. He recommended no chemo and no radiation. The tumors were well contained within the right breast with no lymph node involvement. He was sure the cancer had not moved. He also said that the taking of my left breast was a proactive way of preventing future breast cancer. Our plan is to watch everything careful by having a check up every four to six months or so, getting off the Prempro as well. *I can LIVE with that—literally.*

Dinner tonight, with Jim and Brenda cooking, was a celebration of no need for chemotherapy. *I am so very blessed.*

LOOK AT ME NOW
By Carolyn Salter

Look at me now
Isn't it great?
I've made it past
Cancer's own use by date!
I'm getting well
I'm winning through
Soon I'll be running
Whirling, dancing with you

Back into life
Back into swing
Nothing will stop me
I'll do everything.
Fear can't take hold
I'm being bold!
Look at me now!
Oh, Isn't it great?

May 23

Today is Butch's birthday. I have no gift and no cake and no party planned. I guess we've had other things on our mind!

Without the drain tubes, the fluid is really building in my chest. It feels very tight and painful, to the point of not being able to breathe. I called the emergency number the plastic surgeon's office had given me and reached the Breast Care Center at Regions Hospital in St. Paul. She told me to come in to the ER and she'd see what she could do for me.

She calmed my fears as she explained that this fluid buildup is very common. It is painful, but it is not dangerous. Some women have to have the fluid aspirated three or four times before it stops collecting. It is part of the healing process. She also informed me that some of the women she has treated have been much fuller than I appear to me. Because I had the tissue expanders in, she was a little hesitant to try to aspirate any fluid for fear that she would accidentally puncture an expander. That would mean surgery again to replace the damaged expander. I encouraged her to try, as the pressure seemed so great and I wanted some relief. It was extremely painful as she inserted the needle. In fact, I cried out and the tears began to flow. She immediately stopped and suggested that we wait for a radiologist to do an ultrasound so she would know for sure where the expanders were placed. She also reassured me that it was not life threatening—just uncomfortable. We decided to wait until Tuesday when I'd see the plastic surgeon again and let him draw off the fluid. She suggested warm showers and pain pills to get some relief now. *Being Sunday, Tuesday feels like a long way away at this point in time. Please help me make it, Lord.*

May 25 DAY 37

I guess I complained so much about the drain tubes that they perhaps removed them too quickly. I am retaining quite a bit of fluid around the tissue expanders. It feels very tight and painful. The plastic surgeon used a needle to aspirate the extra fluid and give me some relief. He didn't seem real concerned over the fluid. *Perhaps I'm just being a baby. I can't believe how tight and uncomfortable it feels.* He then began to fill the tissue expanders with saline solution. The valve in the expander was marked with a tiny magnet. The doctor used what looked like a miniature "stud finder." He ran that over my chest to locate the magnet and thus find the valve through which the saline solution was added. My shape is beginning to grow! Pretty amazing stuff.

Bill and Phyllis, good friends of ours, brought dinner this evening. We're going to be pretty spoiled soon when all of this food stops coming! We have some wonderful cooks for friends!

May 26

My Gratitude Group came today and brought such joy. They cleaned my house from top to bottom, washed and ironed clothes, scrubbed floors, cleaned toilets. They brought plants and flowers for me to enjoy. On top of all that, they served lunch and enjoyed it with me and left another meal for dinner that evening. I sat in my lazy boy and cried as I watched my friends cleaning and scrubbing for me. We laughed, cried, prayed, ate and enjoyed being together. It became a grateful celebration of my prognosis and eventual return to good health. *Gratitude in action! What more can I say? It was one of the most memorable days in my life. The feeling of being loved is all around me in the people that continue to minister to me and my daily needs.*

May 27

The fluid continues to gather around the expanders. It was beginning to feel tight again. I called the plastic surgeon's office and was told to come in and have one of his partners draw some of the fluid off to give me relief. It worked. I wonder how long this will continue. *The drain tubes should have been left in longer, I guess. That's my opinion—no one ever said that to me. The tubes were really uncomfortable, and I'm glad they're gone. I'm wondering if I'm going to have to learn to live with this discomfort and tightness the rest of my life.*

May 28

We were planning on heading to Rainy Lake today to open the cabin up for the season. Krisi and Jeff had both taken the day off of work to join us for the weekend. Butch was afraid that the trip would prove to be too much for me. He didn't think I'd be able to sit still and watch everyone else work and that I would overextend and put myself backwards on the healing process. Instead, we took a road trip to Wausaw and Waupaca, Wisconsin, to look at a couple of tractors that Butch had found online. It turned out to be a fun day; a long drive, but fun. The tractor in Waupaca was what Butch was looking for, so he made the deal and came home a pretty happy camper. I didn't do much but ride, eat and sleep. Krisi and Jeff joined us for the day. *It's always good to spend time together.*

May 29

Yesterday's trip tired me out big time. I slept most of the day. The fluid is building again and getting tighter and tighter. They keep telling me this is normal. *I have to take their word for it. I don't like it. I feel like I'm carrying around something big and hard on my chest. My plastic surgeon tells me that I have a vivid imagination. He should try carrying it around for a while. I'm sounding a little crabby today.*

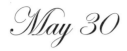 *May 30* DAY 42

    I drove myself to church today. It was good to be back. I received lots of hugs and best wishes. I felt very loved and supported.

    I'm getting pretty full of fluid again. It feels like I have an inner tube around my chest and it is getter tighter and tighter. I'd like to make it until Tuesday's appointment rather than go to Regions Hospital ER on the weekend. I'm learning that the tightness is normal and not to worry about it, just live with it.

May 31 DAY 43

    The weather was pretty rainy and cold. Krisi and I went shopping in Woodbury for her birthday tomorrow. Casual Corner worked out well. We were headed to have our nails done, but the places were all closed for the holiday. In spite of the rain and wind, Butch and Jeff burned a big pile of brush at the farm. We squeezed in a "hotdog burn" between the showers.

I made the holiday weekend without going to the ER to have fluid removed. Carole, my friend, drove me to the clinic today. I feel pretty good, a whole lot stronger. The plastic surgeon drew out more fluid from around both of the expanders. He then put more saline solution into the expanders on each side. My left breast is now 90% full. Next time he'll just put in a little more, then we'll stop. I told him that for forty years I was big breasted and that I did not want that again. As he was filling my right breast like what seemed forever, I said, "Hey, remember I don't want to be a Dolly Parton!" He laughed and said that he was doing a little trick and drawing off some fluid. I was impressed. When he finished, he told me that he felt perhaps my right expander was damaged from all of the aspirating of fluid, which means it may have a hole in it. If so, it will need to be replaced in another forty-five minute surgery to remove the damaged expander and put in a new one. He had me feel how hard my right breast was. He told me that if it gets soft and squishy in the next day or two that we do have a leak. If that's the case, I'm to call immediately and they will get things rolling for surgery so we don't delay the process too much. He was glad that I was feeling so positive about everything and hated to tell me that perhaps we were facing a little setback with a leak. I told him, "I'm this far now and not about to quit. I'll do what I need to do. I don't need chemo or radiation and the cancer is gone. What more can I ask for? If we need to replace the expander, then that's what we'll do. It's not the end of the world."

Carole and I went for coffee before coming home. We stopped at Valley Creek Mall where I picked up two charms for Krisi's birthday today. We'll be celebrating at Wiederholt's Supper Club this evening. I'll try not to think about a possible leak.

June 2

The birthday party was fun last night. The food was great as well. Jeff gave Krisi a gold toe ring as a gift. Her dad asked her, "What the hell is that for?" She just grinned and held the ring up to her nose and laughed. Butch responded, "Oh, for crying out loud!" *We all laughed and it felt so good to feel so normal.* We saw another couple there having a quiet dinner compared to our noisy one. He also is dealing with cancer and not with the glad results that we are experiencing. But for the grace of God go I. We didn't even talk about my squishy right expander.

June 3

I called the plastic surgeon's office today and talked to Barbara. I told her that my right expander had gotten soft. She wasn't surprised. We talked about scheduling surgery. Later in the afternoon she called back with surgery scheduled for Thursday, June 10, at noon, at Lakeview Hospital in Stillwater. I was to arrive at the hospital at 10:00 A.M. I was to come into the clinic on Tuesday, June 8, to see the plastic surgeon before surgery. Here we go again. My positive attitude was leaking into some anger.

June 7

I had another pre-op physical today at the clinic in Stillwater. Some of the tests did not have to be repeated from my last pre-op since it was less than a month ago. That made me feel somewhat better.

June 8

All I do is go to the doctor! Today it is back to the plastic surgeon's office. I wonder how the rest of the world is doing.

June 10   **DAY 53**

I now know the routine. Going in this morning for surgery was certainly not as bad as a month ago. Some of the same people were working and were a little surprised to see me back so soon. This time I walked into surgery and got up on the table before they started to put me under. I really hadn't seen the operating room before. I was much more relaxed. All went well, and by 4:00 P.M. I was home and back in my healing chair with pills for pain and pills to stop any infection. We were back to the drain tube routine as well. The healing should go faster this time.

June 15   **DAY 58**

Back to the clinic again today. During surgery, they started to put saline solution into the expander so that we didn't get too far behind. Healing happens and things look really good. I feel a lot of tightness in my breasts. (I'm beginning to feel like they belong to me and are a part of my body. I can't believe I just called them my breasts!) Sometimes it feels like I have on a new bra that is too tight and itchy and sore. Especially when I'm tired, I get that feeling. I want to take the bra off and get some relief, but it is inside me and cannot be removed. The best remedy is to lie down and stretch out. The plastic surgeon said that all looked great. He added more solution, removed the drain, and told me to come back in a month.

Shortly after my surgery Mickey O'Connor came to visit me. She brought with her a pink Beanie Baby named Hope to help with my healing. She also brought information on a breast cancer support group that meets in Hastings on the third Wednesday of each month at the Regina Care Center. Mickey and her friend, Claire Mathews, lead the group and invited me to join.

This evening at 7:00 was the first meeting that I attended. The women there ranged in age from thirty-two to ninety-three, all of whom had suffered with breast cancer at one point in time. Some were ten-year survivors, some were longer and some were shorter. Some had finished treatment long ago and some were just starting. One gal had just had her surgery the day before I had mine. This was her first time attending as well. The women shared their stories with us and made us feel very welcome. We shared our stories and discussed the many differences and similarities that we found. I can see that we all have a lot to learn from each other and to share with each other and to support each other, which is the purpose of the group.

We talked, laughed, hugged and enjoyed each other's company. They have about thirty women on their membership list with about ten in attendance. I had no idea how prevalent this disease really is. I talked about my feeling that everyone was staring at my chest. Most of the women laughed and began to share with me their "staring at chest" stories. I left the meeting feeling like I belonged. I will return for the next month's meeting.

June 25 DAY 68

Today's checkup was with my internist. It was to see how I was doing with the Paxil and without the Prempro and to check on my blood pressure. I'm experiencing some hot flashes and a few night sweats. That is what the antidepressant is supposed to be helping with now that the Prempro is gone. He wanted to know if the symptoms were unbearable or if I thought I could handle it. When I think about where I've been and how far I've come, I guess I can handle a few hot flashes! I really don't want to take any more pills than necessary. Another good report. We're moving along toward health.

I was complaining to my friend Carole that it seems like all I do is go to the doctor. She replied with a twinkle in her eye, "Well, Diane, don't you know that's what old people do with their time?" *I guess if the shoe fits, wear it! Right?*

June 25-28 DAYS 68-71

Butch's sister, Rita and her husband Joe, along with Joe's brother Mel and Mel's wife Julie, offered to help us open up the cabin for the summer this weekend. We all headed north to Rainy Lake and to our island "Campbellot." It felt so wonderful to be there again. We call it our little bit of heaven on earth. Earlier this spring, I wasn't so sure I'd ever see it again. Thanks to our visitors we accomplished the opening tasks and still had time for a little fun. *What would we do without friends?* I wasn't allowed to do much of anything. I'm going to be spoiled rotten before this cancer journey ends!

I'm becoming more and more comfortable with my new body parts. Sometimes I forget all about them. I suppose it's like wearing braces on your teeth. They are uncomfortable at first, but as time goes on you tend to forget about them, and then they become the norm. Some days I wake up and get out of bed and feel like I'm carrying around a wooden shelf on my chest. My underarms feel better without the drains and all, but they still rub on the fat, or whatever I can feel there. The expanders are getting full and feel pretty hard to me. When I bump into something with my chest, it feels weird and pretty fake. I feel like I have a book strapped to my body, and that is what I hit. When I give people hugs, my new breasts feel hard. *I wonder what they feel like to the person I'm hugging. No one has ever said anything about that, but then I guess they probably wouldn't. I'll have to ask someone sometime.*

Wow! It's the end of June. The time is going. Throughout all of this I've never had that "boobless" feeling. I'm glad that I could start reconstruction immediately and didn't have to experience that flat chestedness. I can look at my body in the mirror and I still have something there. The scars are a badge of courage that I wear proudly. I've even shown them off to my girlfriends occasionally. Most are eager to see and feel. Some turn away. When people ask I'm eager to share, as it helps me as well to talk about it and to be comfortable with it. Krisi was right so many months ago when she told me to come up with some smart remark to break the ice. I usually pull my shirt tight and say something about the new me. That gets people laughing and gives them permission to look and ask questions—which they do, men and women alike. Once that's over, we can get on with the conversation.

I'm beginning to feel more and more like being out and about with family and friends. Walks, lunch dates, a little shopping and cleaning house, as well as cooking and baking, fill my days. I'm so glad to be able to do those things once again.

July 2-5

The Denmark Township Card Club, a group of our friends and neighbors that meets monthly to play cards and talk smart, went with us to Rainy Lake. It was a fun weekend as usual and it felt so good to be both back at the lake and out with friends—back to a more normal life. Of course, I wasn't allowed to do too much of anything in the way of work. What's wrong with that?

July 9-11

We had the Lindemann Family Reunion in Lady Smith, Wisconsin, at Jason and Carie's lodge. With twenty-one of us there, they had room for all. What an amazing place. We had a great time. Matching T-shirts, fun and games, lots of good food. Who could ask for more? Some of the women in the family wanted to have a peek at my new chest, and others did not. I'm comfortable doing that as I do not really feel like it's me. It's recreated, and smaller, with scars running from under my arms to the middle of my chest on each side. It really doesn't look too bad.

My first year of college I went to Mankato State, where I made many wonderful friends. A group of us still get together for lunch now and then to get caught up with each others' lives. Today we met at LeeAnn's in Hastings. The conversation, of course, eventually turned to breast cancer. They had many questions and many fears. We talked for a long time as I explained the procedure I was undergoing to have new breasts reconstructed. I finally asked if they would like to see. Right there in the kitchen I took off my blouse and continued the discussion using my body as a prop. One of the gals laughed and said, "Boy, you can never take the teacher out of Diane. Who else would turn this into a teachable moment?" Another remarked, "I think this is very helpful. Who knows, maybe next week it will be you or I facing the same thing. It's good to know a little about this." It made me feel good to be able to share and perhaps in some way help someone else.

Today's fill at the plastic surgeon's, I think, will be my last. I'm comfortable with the size and feel pretty good about stopping. I've been wearing a sports bra that zips up the front on the advice of my doctor. He felt that the bra would help hold the expanders and push them more towards the front to give me more of a natural look and to help with the discomfort I still feel under my arms. He's right. It has done all of that.

He now wants me to go for a couple of months and in a sense, "test ride" my new breasts. "Try on your clothes and see if you like the look and feel of the way they fit," he told me. He also explained that if I'm not happy, we can easily add more fluid or take some out, depending on what I wanted. He gave me a thirty-page document to read regarding silicone implants and assured me that at my next visit we would discuss the options thoroughly. He wants to wait now for the expanders to do their work and create a pocket for the implants. Then we'll talk about the next surgery.

It certainly feels great to be this far along. Some days I can forget all about it. Only when I take off my shirt am I reminded of my continuing journey. Some days are still uncomfortable physically. If I'm busy and don't think about it, my new breasts feel fine. At other times, I can still feel "the book" I'm carryng out front. That usually happens when I'm tired. I've had a few opportunities to share personally with a couple of women facing breast cancer and surgery. I hope I have been as helpful to them as others were to me.

I attended my second breast cancer support meeting tonight. Many of the same women were there as last month. No one in the group had undergone breast reconstruction. In fact, one of the leaders said that only one other woman in the entire group had had reconstruction. They all wore prosthesis or nothing at all. They had many questions for me. After trying to answer their questions as best I could, I finally said, "Well, would you like to see?" The leader answered for all when she said, "Oh, I was hoping you would say that!" as she quickly jumped up and closed the door. Another one of the gals closed the drapes as she said, "People walking by might wonder what kind of a meeting we are having here." So we had a little show and tell time after which they had more questions. They were all very interested and very grateful for my willingness to share. *Perhaps in this way I may be helping other women make decisions about their own bodies.*

All went well at the plastic surgeon's today. The healing and the stretching are happening. We've stopped adding solution as I feel that I am as large as I would like to be. The doctor reassured me that if I changed my mind, we could always add more. In fact, he also said that if I felt I was too large, solution could be removed. Now we need to wait a couple of months to let nature do its work and form the cavities for the implants. We discussed the pros and cons of saline solution implants and silicone implants. The saline implants, as I understand it, will feel somewhat harder than the silicone. If they develop a leak, the saline solution would be absorbed easily by my body. The solution tends to evaporate slowly from the saline implants, creating the need to replace them in ten to fifteen years. The silicone implants, on the other hand, will have a more natural feel. The silicone tends to adhere to itself. If a leak should develop, the silicone would tend to stay in the cavity created for the implant. Replacement of the silicone implants would be necessary between fifteen to twenty years. Because the silicone is not approved by the FDA, I would need to be a part of a five-year study, which means a yearly visit to the plastic surgeon. Not all surgeons and not all hospitals are approved to insert the silicone implants. My plastic surgeon can do the surgery, but I would need to go to Regions Hospital in St. Paul rather than Lakeview Hospital in Stillwater. I would also have to be registered with the FDA so that they would know how to contact me in the case of a recall. *The more natural feel and the longer time frame before replacement helped me to decide to go with the silicone implants.* I made my decision and signed the necessary paperwork. *It seems like the decisions are getting easier.*

The support group met again tonight. Anne, the girl that had her initial surgery the day before I did, came this evening with a scarf over her head. Her hair is entirely gone from the chemo. She very bravely took off her scarf to show us her bald head. Her goal is to walk into a store without her scarf for the entire world to see. "Look at me. I'm fighting cancer. This is who I am, like it or not!" is the message she wants to give. I told her that I had to stop at Walgreens on my way home and invited her to join me scarfless if she'd like. She declined my offer and said that she wasn't quite ready yet.

I look at Anne and once again realize how grateful I am. I could have been bald by this point and wearing a scarf as well if I would have needed chemotherapy. I admire her courage and strength. What a role model she is for her own daughter and family. Without coming to this support group, I never would have known Anne's story or the stories of all the other women that attend. Knowing them and their stories helps me to know myself better. I thank God for leading me in this direction. This support group thing works for me. I know there are many women out there who do not take advantage of this kind of assistance. I am grateful that it helps give me strength and that I perhaps can help others in the process.

September has been such a busy month. First we went to Mount Pleasant, Iowa, for a Steam Engine Show. Later in the month it was off to Reno for the National Air Races. And finally we headed to our cabin in Canada. Soon we'll be heading back out to the west coast to Sacramento for a family wedding, then back to the cabin to close up for the winter. There just has not been time to schedule in my surgery to have the expanders removed and the implants inserted. I'm now scheduled for surgery on Friday, October 15. The original schedule was for a week earlier on October 8, but the plastic surgeon will be out of town as he's going home for the Canadian Thanksgiving that weekend. His office called and rescheduled for the fifteenth. *I was bummed, but what's another week after I've waited this long?*

I have a pre-op visit with the plastic surgeon this morning at 8:20, then a few weeks to wait and we're home free. Yeah! A little more healing to do and this ordeal is over. Hurrah!

What a disappointing visit that turned out to be! The doctor came in and did his usual exam. We talked about nipple creation. I asked if that happened at this next surgery. He explained that the nipple creation and the tattooing were two separate procedures that would happen down the road a bit yet. That was news to me. I figured this would be the end. He then asked, "Well, what's the plan?"

I said, "What do you mean, what's the plan? I'm scheduled to have my implants inserted on October 15. Don't tell me you're going to postpone again? Won't you be back in town then from your vacation?"

He replied, "Hasn't anyone called you?" He then went on to explain that he was now on probation and would not be able to put in my implants until further notice. I was pretty much blown away. No questions or comments came to my mind. I must have been in a state of shock. His assistant, Joan, told me that it was a paper work mix up and that it would be straightened out soon. She suggested I just be patient and wait for the doctor to do the surgery, as I would be more pleased with the outcome. I left the office totally confused and frustrated. I called Butch from my car and he reminded me that I have every right to have all of my questions answered. He suggested that I call the office again when I get home and find out just exactly what is going on and when the surgery could be scheduled.

We have a neighbor who is a plastic surgeon in Minneapolis. I decided to give him a call to find out just what he knew about this probation business. His wife said she would contact him and have him get back to me. By now, I had quite a few questions on my to-find-out list. *I was beginning to question the integrity and credibility of the plastic surgeon that had been chosen. What's a person to do when you are halfway through the reconstruction process and suddenly your plan no longer exists?*

I called Joan again at the plastic surgeon's office and she reassured me that this probation had nothing to do with his credibility. She explained to me that because I had chosen to have silicone implants, an extra amount of paperwork was required as the silicone is not approved by the FDA. I knew this as I had been given about 30 pages of information to read and sign discussing the risks and all, as well as agreeing to be part of a five-year study because of the silicone. She explained that that was only part of the paperwork. The doctor had more forms to fill out for the facility where the surgery would be performed. The mix up with one or more of these forms was not on my case but with another patient of the doctor. When this happens, the doctor is put on what they call "probation" until the paperwork is straightened out. No other implants can be put in until the probation is lifted. She assured me that everything possible was being done to get this problem taken care of. She felt confident that I would have my surgery on October 15. She promised to call me as soon as she had any news either way.

Later on in the evening our neighbor returned my call. He had talked to my plastic surgeon's office and had been given pretty much the same information as I had been told. He assured me that what I had been told was truthful and that was actually how the system worked when it came to silicone implants. He also helped to relieve my growing anxiety over the capability of my doctor. He said that he had an excellent reputation and was a fine surgeon. He also offered to do the surgery for me if mine was not able to get the problem straightened out. We laughed about how we could meet at the mailbox for my exams. I could just lift my top and he could do the exams under the bright blue sky and the peering eyes of the entire neighborhood. In all seriousness, he felt that it would be best for me to finish up the reconstruction with my original surgeon as he was very capable and had started the procedure and knew me and my circumstances. He assured me that it would all get done, perhaps not within my time frame, but that it would happen.

I continue to ask why this all has to be so difficult. I run and run and then hit another cement wall. I really have tried so hard to keep up with a positive attitude and a sense of humor throughout. It is difficult to understand. However, as my neighber said, it will all happen. Perhaps just not in my time frame. I continue to struggle with my impatience. God in his wisdom must have this lesson for me to learn regarding patience. When I prayed for patience a number of years ago, I found myself teaching first grade. Now that truly is a lesson in practicing being patient. There is a difference, however, in being patient with children and being patient within my own life. I continue to learn and grow.

When I think about this nipple business I ask myself, What do I really need them for? If I have them created, I'll just have to wear clothing that will help to cover them up so they don't show. Why do I even want them? Why don't I just stop at the end of this next surgery? Do I need the tattooing? I don't think so! When discussing this issue with my doctor, he asked me about Krisi and was sure that being a young woman of the 2000s that surely she had a tattoo. I guess he doesn't know Krisi very well! Once again I ask, Why do I need that? I really don't plan on being a topless waitress or anything at this stage in my life. And I don't make it a habit of running around nude. Butch tells me that it's my body and I need to decide what I want and don't want. Another decision to make. At this point in time, I'm thinking NO to both the nipples and the tattooing. I have time to make my final decision one of these days.

September 23

DAY 156

    Joan from the plastic surgeon's office called today to tell me that all was taken care of and that my surgery would go on as scheduled on October 15. She explained that I would receive a mailing with information from Regions Hospital along with a post-op appointment date with the doctor. That information would arrive in a day or two. I'm a happy camper once again.

    I wonder why all the bumps are put in the road? Why can't things go smoothly as planned? Why did I have to endure two more days of frustration before the crooked road was made straight once again? I thank God for the good news of surgery being back on schedule. Now it's on to Sacramento and then closing up the cabin.

116

The trip to California and the wedding all went well. It was especially warm. I expected somewhat cooler temperatures in October. High 80s or low 90s are not my cup of tea. The week in Canada was spectacular—much cooler temperatures, bright sunshine, and beautiful fall foliage. We visited with many friends and buttoned up the cabin for the winter. We came home on Monday so that I could get ready for my surgery on Friday. Today I have my pre-op physical with my internist. I could not get in to see him in Stillwater until after the October 15, but he had an opening today at his Somerset, Wisconsin, office. It was a beautiful day for a drive along the river. Once again I enjoyed God's creation in full fall color.

My physical went well and I even received a flu shot in spite of the shortage of serum this season. I guess that is one advantage to having been diagnosed with cancer this spring. As I was about to leave, my internist told me that I really looked good. He felt that I really looked at peace. He quickly added that he didn't mean that I was off the wall before, but that I now seemed so calm and at ease with this whole thing. I agreed that I did feel that way and contributed the feeling to all of the love and support that I had been given by my family and friends. He especially asked about Butch and wondered how he was doing with the changes in my body and in our life. I told him how lucky and blessed I was. Butch has been my strength, and he is the one that keeps me grounded and gives me a reality check when needed. He then explained that not all husbands handle it that well and reassured me that I indeed was fortunate. We talked about the nipple and tattooing issue as well. He reassured me once again that the decision was totally mine. In a sense, he gave me permission to stop the reconstruction procedure at the point that I felt comfortable with. "Don't be forced into anything that you do not want." *I appreciate his most caring advice. With that physical behind me, the next and hopefully final step is the surgery on Friday.*

I found this poem from Carolyn that puts into words what Butch has said to me through his words, actions, and love.

HEY BABE
By Carolyn Salter

Hey Babe, you're still the one
Cancer doesn't kill off love you know.
And while you don't like your body
I still do.
Even the missing bits
It's all part of you.

Look beyond the physical
Do you think that's all I find?
Look beyond the skin deep
Go into your mind
(It's a great place to be)
There's a whole sea of knowledge there
So don't despair.
Just because we can't do
All we once could
You're still the one for me
Doing me good.

Isn't that weird
I'm learning more from you
Than the other way round.
You're my support.
And I'm glad I've got you, Babe
So glad I've got you, Babe
And my love abounds.

The day is rainy and chilly. I guess it's a good day for surgery. A nice long nap this afternoon in my lazy boy with my favorite quilt and afghan will be just the ticket. We arrived at the hospital at my appointed time, 8:45 A.M. I guess it was more like 9:00 a.m after we drove around the parking ramp at Regions a few times trying to figure out just where to park. No food or drink since midnight last night finds my stomach growling a bit. *I feel pretty calm. Knowing that this is my last big procedure makes me feel good.* We check in at the desk. Butch is given a pager with the instructions that when the doctor is finished and ready to consult with him, the lights will blink.

My name is called and in we go to get ready. I'm instructed to put on my gown, long white stockings to prevent blood clots, and fancy little paper booties that I can't get to stay on my feet. The nurses come in to get my legs wrapped up in funny looking moon boots that go to my knees. Hanging from the bottom of the boots are plug-ins of some sort. Another blood clot prevention device, the nurse tells me. She also gives me a lesson on "Booty Putting On 101" as she quickly puts my feet correctly into the slippers. The next step was the IV. The first attempt in the left arm left me with a real burning feeling as well as swelling and stiffness in my thumb. That one came out quickly with a second try in the right hand that was successful. Now that I'm all hooked up, I need to go to the bathroom, of course. So IV bag and all, off I waddle to the restroom down the hall. Once back in bed, I'm visited by all members of the surgical team. The plastic surgeon draws on my expanded chest all kinds of artwork. Papers are signed and we're ready to go. They come in to tell me that the schedule has been changed from 11:30 to 10:15 A.M. *That is fine with me. I'm ready to go. Let's get this over with.* I can see the team standing around out in the hall waiting for the surgical room to be ready. It's now 10:17 A.M. Then 10:20 A.M. Finally the surgeon comes in with his surgical hat pushed up funny. He has a strange look on his face and my first reaction is, "Oh no! Don't tell me this is not going to happen?"

"That's right!" he replies. "Your implants are in Indianapolis and will not be here today."

"Shit!" was the first expletive out of my mouth.

He went on to explain that "she," whoever she may be, checked the schedule and saw that the surgery for October 8 had been canceled. Not looking ahead to see if it had been rescheduled, "she" sent the implants back to Mentor, the company where they were made. Then he looked at me and said, "Why did you cancel for October 8?"

"I didn't!" I replied. "You did. You were going out of town. Remember? So what happens now? When can we reschedule? When will the implants get here?" My questions went on and on.

He explained that Valerie, his secretary, was working on that right now and would probably have an answer for me before we left the hospital. He walked out of the room shortly thereafter. *I'm sure that somewhere in the conversation he said he was sorry, but the apology does not come to mind.*

Butch and I both looked at each pretty dumbfounded. "Now what do I do?" I said as I pushed the button for the nurse. An aide came in to see what I needed. I told her I needed to go home, so please get someone in here to unhook me. The nurse arrived just as my tears started to flow. She comforted me as best she could and apologized for the mix up. She removed the IV and suggested I take the stockings and boots home and bring them back when the surgery was rescheduled. Butch looked at me pretty incredulously and we pretty much in unison said, "No way! We're not hauling that stuff around. Just throw it away." I dressed in a daze and we walked out of the surgery center. Butch dropped his pager at the desk and we headed silently for home. There didn't seem to be anything to say but, "Can you believe this?" *Another cement wall, and this felt like a pretty big one to me.*

After arriving home, the list of questions began to grow again. I called the surgeon's office where Joan answered and apologized several times. She explained that someone at the hospital had sent the implants back to the manufacturer after seeing that the surgery on

120

October 8 had been canceled. "We don't make these kinds of mistakes often, but when they happen it seems like they happen again and again to the same patient," she offered. I was not comforted. She also went on to say that she thought perhaps early November would be the first time the schedule would allow another surgery. I did not agree with her. She suggested I talk to Valerie, as she's responsible for the scheduling. Valerie apologized at least three times as well and went on to tell me that we were scheduled for Thursday the twenty-first. "Of November?" I snapped. She calmly set me straight and replied, "No, that's next week, Thursday at 7:30 in the morning. I did some juggling around and was able to get you in then, which was the earliest I could do. We'll update your pre-op physical when you arrive at the hospital." "Thank you!" was about all I could manage to respond.

I then sent off the following email to family and friends and hit the couch, where I slept for the rest of the afternoon:

Family & Friends,

It is October 15, 2004, a little after 12:00 P.M. I'm home from the hospital, as my surgery did not happen today. (I'm a little angry—maybe a whole lot angry is better wording.) I arrived at the hospital at my appointed time. We did all the pre-op stuff, including starting the IV (twice—once in each arm!?!?!?). I had talked to everyone I needed to talk to including the surgeon. He marked me all up with his black pen, signed and initialed me and we were just ready to go into the operating room when he came back in to my room and told me that the implants were not there. They had arrived on Tuesday and had been sent back to the company because my surgery on October 8 had been canceled. No one bothered to check to see if it had been rescheduled. So we wasted a lot of time for a lot of people for nothing. So, rather fuming, I dressed and we left. Butch was not a very happy camper either. Now that I've finally had something to eat, I feel a little better. After calling the plastic surgeon's office, I'm rescheduled for Thursday, October 21 at 7:30 in the morning. All I can say is it better work this time or I'll . . . or I'll what? What choice do I have at this point? I'm sorry to say I cried and hollered a bit, but no implants, no surgery. And we trust our lives to the medical system? I wonder! God in His wisdom must have a reason for all of this—but I'll be damned if I can figure it out right now. Thanks for listening. Keep those prayers coming as I'm losing patience.

I still cannot believe it. I figured by now I'd be finished and recovering. I'm angry to say the least, but what can I do about it? Not much. I still need to have these expanders removed and the implants put in. I can not do it myself. No one said it would be easy, but no one said it would be this frustrating either. Valerie in our conversation earlier said, "Well, at least they hadn't put you out yet!" I didn't find that very comforting either, or funny, at this point in time.

Now my schedule is all goofed up. At least I can still host the seminar on Wednesday for my students. I may need to reschedule some of their observations, however, depending on my recovery. It will all work out, but why do I have to make all of the concessions? I guess I'm feeling pretty sorry for Diane right now. I need to remember that things could always be worse. I am still thankful that I did not need to undergo chemo or radiation. I am still thankful that the cancer is now gone from my body. I am still thankful that I have many years of living to look forward to. I am still thankful that I have the support and love of family and friends holding me up through all of this. I just need to continue to work on being patient and resign myself to the fact that I am not in control of these circumstances, but I am in control of my reaction to it. I'll keep working on that with God's help.

I decided that today in church I would make an announcement about my "surgery that didn't happen." That way I'd only have to tell the story once and would have fewer questions after the service. So I stood up at the appointed time and told my tale. I said that I wouldn't repeat what I said when the surgeon came in to tell me that the surgery wasn't going to happen. Obid, our pastor, was quick to say, "What DID you say, Diane?" I waited a few seconds, weighing it over in my mind, and then I shouted, "Shit!" The congregation laughed and broke into applause. *The hugs, kisses and best wishes I received after the service was heartwarming and overwhelming. What do people do without such a community to support them?* My daughter looked at me astonished and said, "I cannot believe you said 'shit' in church!" Then she grinned.

Hopefully my sense of humor about this whole thing is returning. I'm still a bit put out about not being called before arriving at the hospital; however, it is a human institution and therefore mistakes must be expected. I just don't like expecting them to happen to me. Wes, a friend from church, suggested, "Why not try an old pair of socks rolled up—who needs silicone?" My outlook is better now and I pray for forgiveness of my anger. I still do feel that it was justified anger, however. Laughing about the whole mess feels better than crying about it. Now I need to get refocused for surgery on Thursday. I don't plan to leave for the hospital until I know that the implants are there waiting. Another friend quipped, "They just don't have extra boobs laying around, huh?" I guess they don't!

Today's online devotional (daily-devotional@bbs.upperroom.org) used this Bible verse as it's basis: "Forgetting the past and looking forward to what lies ahead, I strain to reach the end of the race and receive the prize for which God, through Christ Jesus, is calling us up to heaven" (Philippians 3:13-14). The mediation talked about Joseph who had many hurts in his life to remember. His brother's threw him in a pit and sold him into slavery. He was slandered by a beautiful woman and thrown into prison. Yet when he came into a position of power in Egypt, he forgave his brothers and he named his son Manasseh, which means "God has caused me to forget" (Genesis 41:51). Joseph shows us how to move forward and forget the hurts of the past.

This "forgive and forget" theme of today's devotional, along with the many emails that I've received the last few days, is certainly my lesson to be learned. Where will it get me to nurse insults and injuries? I have come too far in this battle and have been way too successful to add hard feelings to it now. Help me, Lord, to leave past hurts behind and forgive those who have hurt me.

The following are a few email responses to the postponed surgery:

"Look at your surgery (or lack of in your case) this way. Most people are mad and upset when they have to have surgery, and you got to get mad and upset WHEN YOU DIDN'T HAVE SURGERY. Always have to be different, don't you. All joking aside, I hope everything goes OK for you. Once again, I will think positive and talk to the guy above for a safe and speedy recovery. Take care."

"I can only imagine how distressed you must feel, after all of your emotional and physical preparation for surgery! Maybe, though, God has another plan, and that by delaying the surgery, you will have a better outcome. Maybe, the implants that were sent back were defective, or your surgeon wasn't at his best that day, or… You'll probably never know, but a week isn't too long to wait. You've already done the hard part—the diagnosis and surgery for cancer—so I know, and God knows, that you can get through this, too, with your usual grace and humor! My prayers are with you throughout this ordeal! (Don't be angry at my "silver lining" interpretation of this set back! I'd be just plain mad!)"

"I'm so sorry Diane. I'm with you, screw the medical system. They have me pretty messed up also & I'm more then pissed. I guess we just pray."

"Sorry to hear no new boobs and will keep you in my prayers. I think of you often and all that you've been through and wonder if I could do the same. Good luck on the 21st."

"My heart goes out to you…what a disappointment. I was angry just reading your note. You're right, there was nothing else to do…but the physical, and probably more so, the emotional drain, had to be tough. Our prayers continue for you with a special one on the 21st. Maybe in God's wisdom…they say not to have surgery on a Friday…who knows. God speed and will see you soon!"

"What a bummer!!!! I don't know what else to say!"

I can not dwell on the pain and hurt and frustration of last Friday. It is over and done. The implants were not there so they could not be put into my body. That will happen on next Thursday. I can fume and fuss and create a big stink, and it will get me nowhere but upset, uptight, and angry. Is that how I want to live? By letting go of the anger now, I will be more stress free and relaxed when Thursday comes and the surgery does happen. I don't want to be the "bitch" they have to do the surgery on today. God in His way is showing me

125

the path to follow. Forgive, forget, accept, will make for a happier me in the long run. Thank you, Lord, for showing me the way.

October 19

I called the plastic surgeon's secretary this morning and my IM-PLANTS ARE IN! We are a go for Thursday the twenty-first in the morning at Regions. I asked her if she wanted me to come and hold on to them in my hot little hands until surgery. She didn't laugh but assured me that they would be safe and available on that morning. She explained that the person responsible for the mix up in sending them back really felt bad and was so sorry. *I was really trying to be funny but I guess my comment was not taken that way. I do believe that there were more people upset about last week than just me. I'll have to make my forgiveness known.*

Isaiah 40:31 was the online reading for today. "Those who wait on the LORD will find new strength." Yes, waiting has been the most difficult part of this whole experience. First it was waiting for test results, then waiting to see the surgeon, then waiting for the day of the surgery, then waiting for healing and expanding, then waiting for the implants, then waiting for surgery again. It certainly has been a lesson in developing patience. Once again the devotional seems to have been written for me, especially the comment about life being easier if God acted according to my own timetable! And if I didn't have to wait and everything was going fine, would I feel as much need for prayers and God's guidance? Another lesson for Diane to learn. My experience has taught me many things. The grass is greener, the sky bluer, my love for Butch is stronger and more secure, I know family and friends DO love and support me and that there is life after breast cancer, I know I'm so blessed not to have had chemo or radiation, and I have a very wise and beautiful daughter who loves me very much. I've learned how faithful God is and have been able to find strength in the challenges I've faced. My surgery will be Thursday! I wonder what surprises and exciting challenges lay ahead for me?

October 20   DAY 183

The many angels in our day-to-day life was the theme of the devotional that I read today. I looked up angel in my dictionary and was not surprised to find the meaning to be "a messenger from God." How many of "God's messengers" have been active in my life as a result of this cancer? When I stop to think about it, I am truly amazed. God's messengers in the form of family and friends have brought me words of comfort or challenge just when I needed them most. God's messengers have brought blessings through family and friends, through phone calls, through emails, through health care providers, through members of our congregation, through students at the seminary, and even through strangers. God's angels are all around me! It is my job to have an open mind and heart to be willing to look for them each and every day. They are there!

I've been assured the implants are at the hospital and waiting for me. *I hope so. I don't want a repeat of the last time.*

A young cancer patient talks about her despair over her hair falling out in today's devotional. She realizes that no matter how small or big the problem, God cares and will help. *Once again written just for me, wouldn't you say? Trust God with the details. Okay, God, here we go.*

Butch and I arrived at the hospital at our appointed time. The nurse that called me in reassured me once again that the implants were there and ready. They updated my pre-op physical as promised and I was ready to go. The gal who had mistakenly sent the implants back a week ago had called me yesterday to apologize. She also told me that she would be in to visit me before my surgery. *I was a little nervous about that visit, as I wasn't sure how Butch would react to her. His anger had pretty much matched mine a week ago.* She was nervous when she arrived. She explained once again what had happened and apologized once more, maybe even twice more. She squeezed my hand and wished me luck and was gone. *That took courage. I admire her for owning up to a mistake and then doing something about it. Butch never said a word. He just smiled at me when she left.* Before taking me to surgery, the nurse gave Butch a voucher for the dining room so he could go and have breakfast while he waited. *I thought that was a little odd. It had never happened before.*

The next thing I remember is waking up in recovery. The man next to me was coughing and keeping me awake and all I wanted to do was sleep. The drain tubes were back, but this time only one on each side. I knew the drill and I knew that we could handle it. It took a while for me to become fully awake. I remember having to move into a wheel chair and sitting there for a while as that awful coughing continued. Finally the nurse wheeled me back into another area where Butch was waiting for me. There was also a bouquet of flowers on the windowsill. I thought that was a little strange, as recovery does not usually allow such a thing. In the bouquet was a free parking pass for the ramp. Butch and I laughed about how he should pull it out and stick it in his pocket. We didn't realize that it was meant for us to use. The nurse came in with water for me and told me to just rest and relax as long as I wanted. "When you feel ready, you can get dressed and I'll deliver you to your car. Take your time. There's no hurry." She was in and out several times and offered me something to eat. Butch helped me to struggle into my clothes. This time I remembered to wear something big and baggy that zipped up the front. As the nurse wheeled me out, she handed me the flowers and told me they were a gift from the hospital. *(Perhaps a little guilt on their part? Forgive and forget—right?)* I said my thank yous and we headed for home. Back to the lazy boy and the pillows and the drains and the pain pills and the healing.

Rest and heal. Heal and rest. I've been here before. This time is easier for sure—certainly not the trauma of the first time around. The drains are uncomfortable but so is the tightness of the collecting fluid without them. I have my own little healing corner back and am doing well. The implants already feel softer than the expanders.

On Sunday evening, Krisi & Jeff were here watching TV with us. I stood up to go to the bathroom and left a smear of blood on the white leather sofa that I didn't know about. I undid my shirt and discovered that the tube on my left side had slipped out about five inches. I knew that it wasn't going to work to try and push it back in that far. I called Butch to come and help me. He was waiting for me to call as he had noticed the blood on the sofa. I asked him what he thought, and he suggested that we pull it out the rest of the way. "It's up to you, Diane. I'll do whatever you want." I told him to go ahead and pull it out. I braced for the sting. Surprisingly it slipped right out. There was only about an inch of the tube left in, which accounted for the bloody mess on the sofa. Once we pulled it out, it was fine. No bleeding or leaking or anything. Krisi was probably the most upset, as she had not been around too much before for the drain extravaganza. She thought perhaps we should go to the ER. Tuesday's doctor appointment was soon enough.

I'm truly beginning to feel like my endurance of this cancer storm is coming to an end. It is not easy in the middle of the stormy tribulations to hang on to God and ride it out. "Why" is a word that keeps coming to mind. Why me? Why now? Why was my storm, compared to others around me, an easier storm? Life is good and so is God. I'll probably never have the "whys" answered. I'm so grateful to be where I am. My post-op visit is tomorrow. Doesn't that sound great—POST-OP? Thanks be to God.

Butch woke me up this morning about 7:30 A.M. With the drain tubes and all, I've been having some difficulty sleeping. I'm a side sleeper and the tubes under my arms make that a little uncomfortable. Butch was waiting for me to call Barbara at the plastic surgery clinic to see what time she wanted me to come in. After my splash bath, I gave her a call. She was just ready to call me to see how Sunday had gone. I explained to her about the left tube having fallen out. After a bit of discussion, I decided to go in this morning and have her pull the other tube as well. Then I'd keep my appointment tomorrow morning with the plastic surgeon for my post-op visit. I told her that my left breast was making funny noises. "Oh, you have the squishies!" she giggled, and explained that that, too, shall pass. It is the implants settling in to new surroundings. *Talk about gross! I've certainly passed Breast Cancer Reconstruction 101! What a lot to learn and experience!*

Barbara was pleased with the way everything looked when I arrived at the clinic. She told me that they call the plastic surgeon "Dr. Breast," as he does such an excellent job of creating a good looking set of them. *I must admit, they do look pretty nice. A whole lot smaller than my original homegrown variety! That is good! I'm a little bruised from the liposuction I had done under my arms. (Can you believe I agreed to that? Me, the one who hated everything about plastic surgery, including the word plastic!)* Well, it does feel better, and the "knots" under my arms are gone. *Another lesson learned: Sometimes I do have to listen to what other people tell me. I do not have all the answers even if I would like to think that I do.*

The day went well. It feels so good to have no tubes, no bandages, no knots under the arms. Butch was concerned that I'd do too much today. I didn't get done half of what I wanted to do. I just finished taking a wonderful shower—the first one since surgery last Thursday. It's amazing how great hot water and soap feels. The implants are already much softer than the expanders ever were. I hope that stays that way. Butch said that the plastic surgeon told him that hardness was a sign of infection and that would mean more surgery. Let's hope that doesn't happen.

October 26 DAY 190

I had my post-op appointment with "Dr. Breast" this morning. Barbara assisted him. We explained about the left drain tube coming out on its own. He explained that he had not stitched it in as he had done before, and because of that they sometimes do fall out. He was not at all concerned. He removed the liposuction stitches and wanted to know if we had accomplished everything in surgery that I wanted done. We discussed a little that my left breast appeared to be a little lower than the right. He assured me that we could fix that fairly easily down the road. We also talked about the softness of the implants compared to the expanders. He explained that they should stay this way but that we wouldn't really know for about six months. My body needs to react to the implants, and we have no way of knowing what that reaction may be. It may choose to make a capsule of hard scar tissue around it or it may not. Time will tell. If the scar tissue forms, there is a surgical procedure to help break up the scars and soften the appearance. "Hopefully that will not happen. And if it does, we'll talk about it then," was his reply. My next appointment is three weeks from now. He encouraged me to return to normal activity but to not take part in sports, jogging, aerobics, and so on, for a few weeks. I agreed that that would be real easy for me to give up!

As he was leaving the room, I told him that I was planning on writing a book about my breast cancer journey. He came back in grinning as I assured him that he would be a part of it. "The final chapter isn't written yet," he cautioned. *See, I do need to continue my work on patience. The doctor has been a constant reminder to me to slow down and take one step at a time. I'm trying. I always want to get from "there to here" yesterday. It feels so good to be on this side of things. I know that I'm not finished with this journey, but it feels good to celebrate the place I'm at today. And I think that is okay! A speaker I attended today said that before you can do anything you have to get up. If you stumble, get up again. Keep getting up until you accomplish whatever it is you set out to do. The next step is to be grateful for steps taken and to express that gratitude. Thank you, Lord, that I am this far on my journey. Be with me as I continue on. Amen.*

I've had a pretty busy week with student teachers and meetings and so forth. It does feel good to be home today with nothing on my agenda. I'm learning that there is nothing wrong with taking a good nap now and then, and that's exactly what I have planned for this afternoon. I'm reading a good book. Talk about a perfect recipe: one good book, one comfy sofa, one fluffy pillow, one soft afghan. Add to that one tired body. Mix together for at least three hours and voila! A little R&R for Diane.

Sometime throughout this journey, I've misplaced a favorite tablecloth. In an effort to find it, I cleaned (and I mean cleaned) two closets today with no luck. As I was finishing up and putting things away, I started with a little itching around my new implants. I put on a little Neosporin and tried to forget about it. We had dinner out with Grandma, Krisi, and Jeff, and as the dinner continued, so did the itching. It was driving me pretty much wild by the time we got home. I added more cream and tried to sleep. After finishing up reading my novel at about 1:30 A.M., I tried the sleep thing again and was at last successful. *Of course my mind is running away with things, and all sorts of bad scenarios arise. What if I'm allergic to the silicone and the implants need to be removed? What if there is a silicone leak and that is what is causing the itching? What if...What if... What if...You know how the brain works at 3:00 in the morning!*

The itching continued throughout the night. With nothing again on my agenda, I decided to sleep as long as possible. The old brain kicks in about 8:30 A.M. with some more of those "what ifs..."

I decided to call the emergency number at Regions to get some advice. Before calling, I took a good look at my chest. The red itching spots followed straight lines along the incisions. It looks to me like I'm having an allergic reaction to the adhesive used in the bandaging. I still called to find out what to do with all this itching. I talked to the on-call physician. He recommended that I use a hydrocortisone cream, rub it well, and take Benedryl. He also suggested that I get in to see my plastic surgeon this week if at all possible just because that would probably make me feel better. He assured me that if I was having a reaction to the implants there would be fever and redness, not just redness following the adhesive line. *That made me much more comfortable. I followed his advice throughout the day and did find some relief.*

As a patient, I have learned that I have every right to ask questions and to get answers for those questions. The old Diane would not want to have bothered anyone and probably would not have called Regions Emergency. But this new, updated model called as soon as she got out of bed today.

A week or so ago, Obid asked me if I would be willing to share my "faith story" at our new celebration service at church today. I did pretty well until I got to the last few pages, when I'm talking about everything that was done for me by my "earth angels." I looked up and half of the congregation was crying, and that did me in. By the time I finished, I think most everyone were crying. Many of them were my "earth angels." Here is my story:

When Obid asked me last week to give my faith story today, he also wisely added, "Make it 10 to 15 minutes." Butch, my husband, tells me that I need grease fittings in my jaws to keep them in working order. Go figure, huh? So with only 10-15 minutes, I decided to talk about my faith story through my recent breast cancer experience, in the hope that my story will be of help to any of you facing troubles of any sort in your life. My story, as you know, has a happy ending. My cancer is gone, no chemo or radiation was needed, just some very radical surgery. Not all stories turn out this way as we all know. I'm very blessed and very grateful. God sent many "earth angels" to care for me—but I'm getting ahead of my story…

Way back a hundred years ago when I was confirmed, our minister assigned me this Bible verse from Psalm 46:1, "God is our refuge and strength, always ready to help in times of trouble." My fifteen-year-old brain couldn't get around that one at the time. I was offended to think that he thought I was going to be in trouble a lot in my life. My fifty-six-year-old brain tells me that he was a very wise man. Age and life experience have taught me that this verse was for me a compliment of the highest form. His belief was that my faith was strong enough to see me through the troubles that I, as well as everyone else, were destined to face in our lifetime.

"God is our refuge and strength, always ready to help in times of trouble. So we will not fear, even if earthquakes come and the mountains crumble into the sea. Let the oceans roar and foam. Let the mountains tremble as the waters surge!" (Psalm 46: 1-3).

My earth began to shake and change and the mountains tremble when my breast cancer "trouble" began in October of 2003. I went in for my yearly mammogram and was called back two days later as some calcifications were found on my right breast. It was decided that an attitude of "Let's keep a close eye on this for six months" would be in order. I made the appointment for April 19—six months to the day—to have a magnification type of screening done. I put it totally out of my mind for five and a half months. Then as the date was nearing I noticed in the mirror that my right nipple seemed to be about an inch lower than my left and that the right breast appeared somewhat larger. Then I remembered my mom telling me after her mastectomy, that she had watched her breast grow and change until she couldn't stand it any longer, so she went to see her doctor. I pretty much froze with the realization of what I was now seeing on my own body.

On April 19 I found myself strangely calm. I had been asking God to give me strength to face whatever was ahead for me. Philippians 4:6-7 came to mind: "Don't worry about anything; instead, pray about everything. Tell God what you need, and thank him for all he has done. If you do this, you will experience God's peace, which is far more wonderful than the human mind can understand. His peace will guard your hearts and minds as you live in Christ Jesus." The peace of God was with me at this moment but would waver as the roller coaster ride of breast cancer was about to take over my life. After the magnification type of screening was over, it took about ten minutes for the doctor to come in to tell me

137

that I was looking at a twenty percent chance of what they saw being malignant. I told him about my mother. He then explained that on a scale from one to five, one being benign and five being malignant, I was about a three. I'm no math whiz, but I think my odds just changed rather quickly. The biopsy was scheduled for April 22. The days leading up to that were filled with fear, tears, love, prayers and a whole lot of work. I pressure-washed the deck as well as all of the deck furniture. I washed windows, moved plants from one garden to another, cleaned my house from top to bottom—anything to keep from thinking.

As hard as I tried to make it all go away and as hard as I tried to go back in time before this all started, it was not possible. I knew where I was and where I wanted to be, and the only way to get there was to travel straight through what ever lie ahead. To get from there to here, I had to take the journey. April 22 dawned with the next step—the biopsy. As I walked into the hospital that morning, I knew that this was just the beginning of many hospital and doctor visits. I had a premonition that malignancy would be found. Where now was the peace of God I had prayed for?

The actual biopsy took quite a long time as I had two areas that needed to be looked at. As I lay on my stomach in a rather awkward position on a very strange table, I recited over and over in my head every Bible verse, prayer, and hymn that I could bring to mind. Remembering the peace that the twenty-third Psalm brought to Sharon Ewald (a member of our congregation who died a few years ago of cancer), I said it over and over and over until the procedure ended.

Now the waiting for results began. I was told it took forty-eight hours to run the necessary tests on the tissue taken. However, since it was Thursday, it would probably be Monday before I would have the results. The weekend brought lots of phone calls and emails from family and friends. They couldn't take the threat of cancer away but they could give me their love and support, so I didn't feel so all alone. Butch, Krisi and Jeff provided that same love and support as well.

The waiting continued…the days slowly passed by. I worried, I fretted, I cried, I prayed and my family suffered along with me every step of the way. No news on Monday. The waiting continued…

My journal entry on Tuesday reads, and I quote, *"The Psalmist wrote, 'Turn to me and have mercy on me, for I am alone and in deep distress. My problems go from bad to worse. Oh, save me from them all!' (Psalm 25:16-17). This is the Daily Guideposts reading for today. Even though I still have not heard my results, I've decided that enough is enough. I'm choosing to live my life as the true gift it is and not obsess and continue to worry over whatever it is in my breast. I will know when I'm supposed to know and will handle it at that time. I've wasted too many days being overly concerned regarding this issue. It's hurting me and my family way too much, and it is time to move on.*

So here we are. Tuesday morning and my life must go on. I encouraged both Butch & Krisi to go to work. They listened to me and decided to do just that. I have more energy than I've had for the last week. The sun is shining and I want to get out in my gardens. The weeds are already getting ahead of me. I know that whatever the results bring, we will be able to handle the days ahead. I have the love and support of family and friends and with God beside me I will make it. Perhaps this is my lesson—perhaps this is where I needed to arrive on my journey through this trial."

Finally on Wednesday morning my gynecologist called with the results. A few days later than I was told I would have the results, wouldn't you say? Breast cancer was definitely confirmed. She had taken the liberty of setting up an appointment for me with a breast cancer specialist and surgeon that very afternoon. Can you say, mastectomy? It is a very harsh word when you are talking about your own body. We left the surgeon's office with pamphlets, appointments, and books. I now knew what I was facing and that I had some huge decisions to make with the help of God and my family. Psalm 46:1 popped into my head again, "God is our refuge and strength, always ready to help in times of trouble." Surgery was scheduled for May 13. Anger swelled within me. Why me, God? Why now? I don't have time to deal with this at this point in my life. I don't want my life disrupted with doctor appointments and all that goes along with it. The anger became so great that I even called my plastic surgeon a donkey (well, that's not the word I used, but you get the point) on our first meeting. I was extremely rude. His office was the last place in the world that I wanted to be. I hate plastic flowers, let alone plastic body parts.

In spite of my attitude, the "earth angels" continued to minister to me. I could see and feel God's hand everywhere. I would be in the midst of making decisions regarding the upcoming surgery…Do I have them take only the breast with cancer, or do I have both breasts taken? Do I need or want reconstruction? Can I have reconstruction started the same day? The telephone would ring and a nurse or doctor or a breast cancer survivor would be on the other end, ready to listen and or share their experiences and cry with me. I'm serving on the Board of United Theological Seminary. The chairman of the committee I've been assigned to called and shared her breast cancer story with me. She told me that my job for the next several months was survival. Now, was that the hand of God, or what? I had no idea she was a survivor before that point. Bryan Olson, our youth pastor, emailed me and asked for my permission to have my name and circumstances lifted in prayer throughout the seminary community. My response was, "Yes, of course. How many women in my situation have an entire seminary praying for them? It certainly won't hurt." Angels in the form of Obid and Margo came to visit, as well as sisters-in-law and sisters in spirit and friends and neighbors.

Butch and Krisi were ever-present angels that held me, cried with me, and loved me.

Decisions were made. Surgery happened and the healing of body, soul and mind began. And still the angels came. Butch and I joked about the delivery trucks backing in and out of our driveway on the Saturday I came home from the hospital. Flowers filled my living room. I told Butch that it smelled like a funeral home in our house. He assured me that it was better than a funeral home, as I was alive and could enjoy the fragrance and beauty of the bouquets and arrangements! Others sent cards and still others brought food. Others made phone calls and sent emails and still others supported Butch and Krisi in ways I don't even know. Angels ministered to me through the music of Don Moen and his music CD, *God Will Make a Way*, as did the poetry of Carolyn Salter and the Breast Cancer Support Group in Hastings. Others came and vacuumed, ironed, dusted and scrubbed. Some sent bracelets. Others drove me to my many appointments. Others sent gifts of books, chocolate, wine and comfy pajamas. The flow of love and strength and healing continued. Prayers were being said for me from coast to coast, as well as in Canada and Australia. Prayer does make a difference, folks. Prayer and love lifted me and carried me through my journey from there to here. I thank you again, my dear "earth angels," for whatever part you played in making that happen for me.

I've learned many lessons throughout this experience:

1. It's God's timetable, not mine.
2. Prayer works.
3. I am loved deeply by many, especially Butch & Krisi.
4. Life is good. The trees are greener and the sky bluer on this side of cancer.
5. Life is too precious to waste and too short to worry over the little things.
6. Choose gratitude—it's a better attitude.

I'd like to close with two poems from Carolyn Salter. Carolyn is a friend of mine that lives in Walcha, NSW, Australia. She lost her brother and mother to cancer and a son to a crop dusting accident. She is highly involved in Australian Relay for Life cancer research fundraising. These two poems are from her book entitled *Hurdles Are For Jumping* that was written especially for the Relay for Life event in her community.

LIFE WAS SO EASY

Life was oh so easy
How could I then know
That this was a path
Down which I would have to go?
No options for me
Journeying with dread
Heavy, awful, arduous,
The path that I must tread.

How could I then know
How much that I would learn?
And the friends that I would make
Who would with each other turn
The negatives to positives
Finding easier ways
Trusting in each other
To lighten heavy, difficult days.

How could I then know
How my perspective would change?
And see my life go right way up
Drastically rearrange.

Life's noticeably different now
Little things become so dear
Troubles once insurmountable
Much simpler now, and clear.

Could I even thank
This strange experience I had?
Will you think me crazy
When I say that I am glad
That this cancer came along
To wake up my whole world?

And now I'm navigating life
With every sail unfurled.

THANK YOU

Thank you for this wonderful day
Thank you for science
The doctors and nurses
Committed to cure.

Thank you
For simple sunshine
For birds
Crashing waves
White laced on a turquoise sea
For sunsets
Sunrises
And flowers.

Thank you
For the universe

I marvel at its enormity
And tiny ants
Wondering if they see me as huge
In their world.

Thank you for family
And friends
More precious than any jewels
Thank you
For another opportunity
But most of all
Thank you
For life.

Amen.

It felt good to share this story today with people that I've known all of my life. Perhaps it is part of the healing process for me, and I did get to thank again so many of my "earth angels" publicly in that way. I had hoped not to cry, but I guess that wasn't possible with so many close friends and family in the congregation. My hope was to help others that are in the midst of turmoil and strife. I received a lot of hugs and positive feedback as I left the church. I guess we really never know how our words affect others.

I had my three-week-after-surgery checkup today with the plastic surgeon. He said that everything looks really good. He removed a couple of stitches that were sticking out. The scars are healing nicely, but he suggested that I use a silicon product to help reduce the redness of the scars and keep them soft. Also in an effort to keep things soft, he demonstrated for me some exercises to use with my new breasts on a twice-daily basis. It's just pushing the implants up and holding for thirty seconds, pushing them toward the center and holding, and pushing them outward and holding again for thirty seconds. That way my body will hopefully not make a stiff or hard cavity around the implants and they will remain more pliable in nature. He said he would see me in one month and at that time we would talk about nipple reconstruction.

I'm seriously thinking about not going any further with the reconstruction stuff. I'm very happy where things are now. I do not wear a bra of any sort and I'm very comfortable. If I have nipples created, I'd only have to wear a bra to cover them up. So why do it? I am so happy to be on this side of things at this point. I really don't want any more surgery for a while. I'll listen to what he has to say because information is good, but I'm leaning at this time towards no nipples. We'll see.

I could not find the product that the plastic surgeon suggested, but I did find something called Scar Therapy that works the same way as he described. The medication is on an adhesive strip that you wear over the scar area for twenty-four hours. Then you change the strip and continue on for approximately eight weeks, at which time you will see a softening of the scar area and a fading of the redness. *It's worth a try. A little expensive, but what isn't that works?*

I'm concerned that my implants may be moving under my arms more, as I seem to be able to feel them more with my arms at my sides. I've been shopping for a bra with a wide band that would help hold in my sides and feel better to my underarms.

Shopping has not been easy. First of all, it is difficult to find a 38 A or B cup that has a wide band on the sides. My fat hangs over the narrow little bands and does not look or feel very great. Size 40 does not come in an A cup. To add to the difficulty, not all brands have the same size cups. They all need to be tried on for proper fit. Yesterday afternoon I tried on every style bra in Herbergers but found none that fit. Either the A cup was too small or the B cup was just a little too big. It seemed to bunch up in the middle with a wrinkle and not lie flat.

I tried again this afternoon at Marshall Field's in Minneapolis. I ended up with a Champion brand bra made for more casual wear. The B cup was again a little too roomy. Maybe if I wash it in hot water and dry it in the dryer it will fit better.

Krisi and I were shopping again and she observed, "Whoever thought, Mom, that you would be looking for an A cup!" Such a problem to have! I guess I'll just go braless. I'll have to ask the plastic surgeon about this next week at our appointment.

I have another check up with the plastic surgeon this morning. Everything is going fine. My left breast is somewhat softer than the right. The scar and everything on the right looks and feels more constricted for some reason. The doctor thought perhaps the extra surgery replacing the damaged tissue expander might be the cause. He didn't seem too concerned about it. He said that everything looked great and that he would see me again in two months, and then after that, once a year to fulfill the requirements of the silicone implant study. Nipple reconstruction and the tattooing will be discussed at that next appointment.

I asked about wearing a bra and whether or not he thought that would be necessary. My concern was that the implants might start floating around and wind up on my shoulder or under my arms. He grinned and assured me that would not happen. I explained how one of my friend's implants had moved higher on her chest. He felt that was a mistake made when the implant was first put into the body. The muscle had not been expanded enough before the implant surgery and therefore allowed the implant to move. In answer to my question about the bra, he told me that at first it is not advisable. The implant needs to settle in and allow gravity to do its work. The implant sags and pulls down to make the breast appear more natural and not so round. Wearing a bra at first can cause the implant to become more shaped like the bra with less of a natural look.

In spite of what he says, I still feel a little more comfortable wearing a bra, as it holds in the fat more under my arms. That underarm stuff has been a problem for me all along. I just don't like the feel of my arms rubbing against that part of my body. It feels like I have too much in the way. I had the same problem with my natural breasts, and wearing a bra made me feel better. I will, however, follow his advice and not start wearing a bra just yet. His nurse didn't think that at this point it would make too much of a difference. She encouraged me to do whatever I was most comfortable with. I've trusted his advice so far, and so far he has been right.

I was busy on my computer today when the dog started making a fuss barking and growling. Then I heard a knock at the door. Our friend, Jim, who was a neighbor and moved to Cloquet, Minnesota, a number of years ago, was at the door. He stepped inside and folded me into his arms with a huge hug. We hadn't seen him since my initial surgery. He recently had undergone some heart surgery himself. I stepped back from his hug and pulled my sweatshirt tight around my body and made some remark about the "new" me. His reply was instant, "You haven't changed a bit. You are still the Diane that we know and love. You are not a pair of breasts. You are still you and always will be. The rest of that does not matter at all, and don't ever forget it!"

Wow! Quite an affirmation from a man's man! He certainly made my day. Many of Butch's male friends, the ones I do not know real well, are now beginning to talk to me about my surgery and all that followed. I guess it took them the six to seven months to feel comfortable doing so. Our close friends, male and female, had no problem supporting me immediately. I took my daughter's wise advice back at the beginning of this, when I was sure no one would look me in the face anymore but would instead be looking at my breasts. She counseled me to come up with some kind of a wise remark that would cause some laughter and break the ice. It worked. It showed people that I was comfortable with my body and that they should be, too, and that it was okay to talk and ask questions. Hopefully I've been able to help people understand breast cancer and the reconstruction process through my willingness to share. It is also very healing for me to do.

Our Breast Cancer Support Group decided to start meeting on the first Wednesday of each month in the morning at a local coffee house in addition to our regular meeting on the third Wednesday evening of each month. We decided this for a few reasons. First of all, we enjoy one another's company. Secondly, it seems like a long time between meetings if you are feeling the need for help, support and camaraderie. Thirdly, some women do not like to drive after dark and find the morning time much easier for them to be a part of the group.

Today was the first of these new coffee meetings and we had a pretty good turnout. Some of the women came and went as their schedules allowed. We laughed, talked, listened and shared for about two hours. Anne, the youngest member of our group, brought a framed postcard that she has hanging in her bedroom. The picture is of a nude woman who has had a mastectomy of her right breast. She is standing tall in the wilderness with her arms outstretched to the sky and a confident smile on her face as she gazes upward. Her body is strong and healthy as she reaches toward heaven. Where her breast had been is a beautiful tattoo of a vine covering the scar. She is called the "Warrior." Anne explained how the picture has been instrumental in giving her hope and courage as she continues her journey with breast cancer. She finds comfort in the strength that the woman portrays and uses her as a role model to emulate.

Each of the women in this group has their own story of their battle. They are all strong, loving, caring women, with much to give and much to teach to those around them. I'm so glad that Mickey, one of the group leaders, invited me to join.

I met with the plastic surgeon this morning for my regular checkup and a consultation regarding nipple reconstruction and tattooing. My left breast is slightly lower than my right. We talked about how he could do a little nipping and tucking to bring it up and make them more even. After giving it a little thought and realizing it would mean more surgery, even though only minor, I declined. I never was perfectly symmetrical before, so why should I want to be now? I'm happy and braless and most comfortable.

The nipple reconstruction would also be just a minor surgery. He would use local anesthesia and something else to relax me and hopefully put me out. The incision would be made along the existing scar, where he would make two flaps of skin that could be brought up and sewn together to make the nipple. The size of the incisions would depend upon how upright I would want the nipples to be. The tattooing would happen two to three weeks later to add the color around the nipple area, creating the areola. As usual, his explanations were very thorough, and he was most patient to answer all of my questions. My decision was not to have the nipple reconstruction done. If I were younger, I perhaps would have given this option more thought. However, Butch assures me that he is happy just having me here and healthy. I'm happy being here and healthy, so for the time being, the answer is no. If I change my mind, this surgery can be done at any time in the future.

I said my good-byes for now as I do not need to return again until the one -year anniversary of my initial surgery. Each year for five years I will need to make that visit to fulfill the requirements of the silicone study that I needed to be a part of in order to have the implants. They assured me that I should call at any time if I have questions or concerns. *Wow! I can't believe I'm here! Is the nightmare really over for now? Is everything really done? Will I be okay without these visits? Thank you, God. Let's get on with life!*

This journey that started last April has now occupied ten months of my life. Standing "here" and looking back to "there," the time seems to have flown. I couldn't have said that in April, as looking ahead for ten months seemed like an eternity. It is funny how time works in that way. It has been a long, arduous, life-changing journey, and yet it only took ten months! The lessons I have learned and the alterations to my body, mind and soul have been transformational, and yet it only took ten months. I am comfortable with my new body. I can look at my new breasts with their fading red, purple and white scars crossing each horizontally, and see beauty and fresh new life. I'm proud of them and the courage they stand for. I see myself as a warrior and I have the scars to prove it, and yet it only took ten months. I'm still too chicken to have my ears pierced, but I made the decision to have both of my breasts removed in order to save my life. Will the cancer reappear? No one has the privilege of knowing that answer this side of heaven. I do know that if it does reappear I have the strength, love, support, and fortitude to face the battle, which only took ten months to prove to myself. I've made the journey from "there" to "here." I'm different than I was ten months ago. I'm thankful for the journey and for those yet to come. Without this journey, would there have been any more journeys to look forward to in the future?

THE SURVIVOR
By Carolyn Salter

I have beaten it
It has gone
No more cancer for me
I'm a lucky one
Mine has been cured
Did I do something differently
From those who did not survive?
Is life really
A huge lottery

With God plucking us
Like weeds
To go or to stay?
If so
Am I a flower or a weed?
Which is which?
Does it matter?
I am alive
I am well
I will live this life
Fully
With thanks.
But at the end
I will have
More questions
Many more questions.

CURED OF CANCER
By Carolyn Salter

Cured of cancer!
Another go at life
When it could have been
So different.
Another chance to live my best
And the best is yet to come.
For I have looked at death
And found it
Not frightening
Surprisingly, not frightening.
Merely sadness at the thought
Of leaving those I love
Of leaving all that is familiar.

But death itself.
No
Perhaps merely the method of death
I wish I could choose.
But slipping the confines of a used-up body
To fly free
To return to the Source
That almost entrances me
Exhilarating thought.

I WONDER
By Carolyn Salter

I wonder if I did choose this
If I thought I would gain
Grow
With this experience
Learn, develop
Evolve into a higher soul
Soar.
Closer to perfection.
Then
When I could not know of human pain
Of the wrench
Desolation
Contemplating the possibility
Of leaving this earth.
Of leaving the love of human family
Such love.

Did I choose this then?
When I was still with God
And knew I would return.

And did He say
This will be hard
But I will be with you?

And did I forget all
When I came here
Struggling to make sense of it
Remembering only vaguely
Vaguely a purpose
A conviction that there was
More to do
More ways to grow.
But how, what was it?
And have I found it now?
Have I followed my path?
Am I fulfilling my dreams
Of long ago
Before I was?
And, if so
Is He pleased?

In spite of my weaknesses and impatience, God's grace has seen me through this breast cancer journey. I am eternally grateful and I will strive "to do more and do better"! Praise be to God!

Part Three

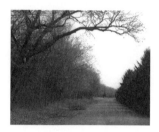

Resources For More Help

Along my journey *From There to Here*, I have found and have been given many resources that were of tremendous help to me. I've included them here so you will not have to search too far for them yourself. They are divided into two sections: Medical Information, and Inspiration and Support. My hope is that they will be of assistance to you in your journey or in your ministry of helping others.

Medical Information

Books
Friedewald, Vincent, M.D., and Buzdar, Aman, M.D. Ask the Doctor: Breast Cancer. Kansas City: Andrews and McMeel, 1997.

Pamphlets
"Breast Cancer Dictionary" (No. 4675-CC). American Cancer Society, www.cancer.org.

"Breast Reconstruction Following Breast Removal." Arlington Heights: American Society of Plastic Surgeons, www.plasticsurgery. org.

"Breast Surgery: From Biopsy to Reconstruction." Krames Communications.

"Mastectomy: A Patient Guide" (97-75M-No. 4600-CC). American Cancer Society, www.cancer.org, 1997.

"Reach for Recovery: Exercises After Breast Surgery" (98-20M-No. 4668-CC). American Cancer Society, 1998.

"Reach for Recovery: Breast Prosthesis Shopping List" (MW531.5), American Cancer Society, www.cancer.org, 2001.

"Taking Time: Support for People With Cancer and the People Who Care About Them" (NIH Publication No. 97-20599). National Cancer Institute, 1997.

Inspiration And Support

Books

Canfield, Jack. Chicken Soup for the Surviving Soul : 101 Healing Stories About Those Who Have Survived Cancer. Deerfield Beach: Health Communications, Inc., www.hci-online.com or www.chickensoup.com, 1996.

Daily Guideposts 2004. Caramel: Guideposts Books & Media Division, www.guideposts.com.

Daily Guideposts 2005. Caramel: Guideposts Books & Media Division, www.guideposts.com.

Salter, Carolyn. Hurdles Are for Jumping: Perceptions of Cancer. Walcha: 2003. (You can order this book directly through Carolyn at: Carolyn Salter, "Wanderriby," Walcha, NSW 2354, Australia. Phone: int + 61 2 67776566; fax: int + 61 2 67776567. Email: dcsalter@northnet.com.au).

Salter, Carolyn. Once Upon A Shooting Star. Henley Beach: Seaview Press, 2002. (You can order this book directly through Carolyn at: Carolyn Salter, "Wanderriby," Walcha, NSW 2354, Australia. Phone: int + 61 2 67776566; fax: int + 61 2 67776567. Email: dcsalter@northnet.com.au).

Williamson, Marianne. Illuminata: Thoughts Prayers, Rites of Passage. New York: Random House, 1994.

Wright, Carolyn Shores. Beneath His Wings, Abiding in God's Comfort and Love. Eugene: Harvest House Publishers.

Music Cds

Moen, Don. God Will Make a Way. www.integritymusic.com
Moen, Don. I Will Sing. www.integritymusic.com

Order Form

Please copy this page, add the necessary information, and mail it with your check or money order, payable to Diane Davies to:

Diane Davies
8487 Quant Av S
Hastings MN 55033

Note: Ten percent of the proceeds from the sale of each book will be donated to the American Cancer Society.

ISBN: 1-930374-18-6
From There To Here $17.00 each   Qty. _____

Total: _____

MN residents add 6.5% sales tax ($1.11/book)   _____

Shipping: $3.00 first book, $1.50 each additional   _____

Total enclosed: _____

Name: _____

Address: _____

City: _____   State: _____ Zip: _____

Phone: (__) _____ Email:_____

You can also order this book securely from DeForest Press at www.DeForestPress.com, or by calling toll-free 1-877-441-9733.